Alternatives to Surrender

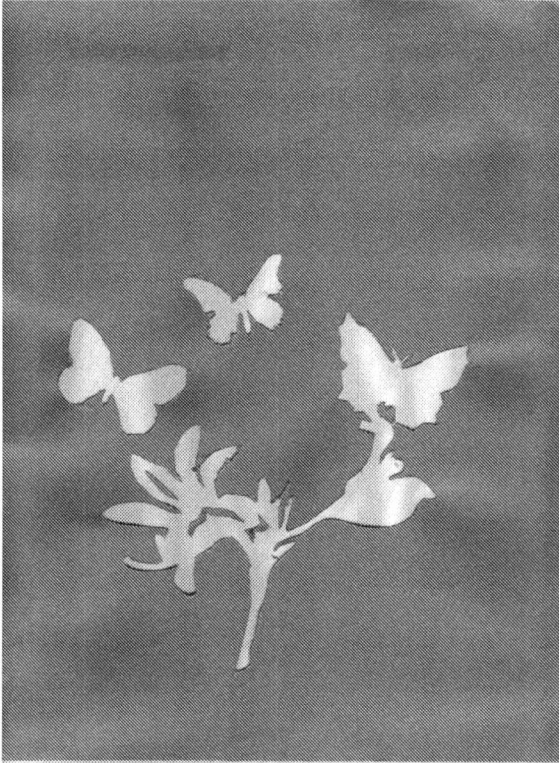

Poems that deal with cancer, survival from cancer,
death from cancer, with loss and recovery

Edited By

Martin Willitts, Jr.

Plain View Press
P. O. 42255
Austin, TX 78704

plainviewpress.net
sb@plainviewpress.net
1-512-441-2452

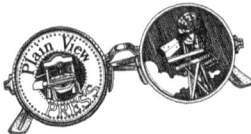

Cover art by: Martin Willitts, Jr. "Resurrection Lily and Butterflies"

(Resurrection Lily (Lycora squamigera) with Magnificent Owl butterfly (Caligo arteus) from Central America on the left, Blue Morpho butterfly (Morpho peleides) from South America in the middle, and Purple Emperor (Apatura iris) from England touching the flower.)

We have two options, medically and emotionally:
give up, or Fight Like Hell.
Lance Armstrong

This project was an individual artist grant funded by the New York State Council on the Arts, and sponsored by Chenango County Council of the Arts.

Acknowledgments:

Christine Orchanian Adler —"Unearthed," *Literarymama. com*; **Sally Bellerose**: "Bye Bye Barbara," Sojourner; *Sojourner, A feminist Anthology*, (*University of Illinois Press*, 2004.) (Reprint); **Gary Blankenship**— "Poetic States VII — Delaware," *A River Transformed*; **Barbara Daniels**: "The Cancer Patient Addresses Her Husband," *25: Women's Perspectives*; "Periwinkle," *Drexel Online Journal, Art in the Air* (reprinted), and "Begging," *bma*; **Maryanne Hannan**: "Change," *Poet Lore*; **Laura Heidy**— "In Utero," *Sol Magazine, Solares Hill Newspaper* (reprinted), and *Poet's Corner* (reprinted); **Joy Harold Helsing**— "Mastectomy," *Brevities*; "Remission," *The Lyric* and *Oncolink.* (reprinted); "The Knife," *Oncolink*; **William Heyen**— "The Matrix," *Pterodactyl Rose*, (*Time Being Books*, 1991); "Strawberries," *The Rope: poems*, (*Mammoth Books*, 2003); **Karla Huston**— "Pencil Test," *Pearl*, *Silt Reader* (reprinted), *Pencil Test*, (*Cassandra Press*), and in the chapbook *Flight Patterns* (winner of the 2003 *Main Street Rag Chapbook Contest*); **Roy Jacobstein**— "Parting Conversation" *Ripe*; **Liz Rosenberg**— "The Blue-Flowered Bell," "The Suffering," and "Because I Was Dying," Children Of Paradise, (*U of Pittsburgh*, 1994); "Valentine's Day At Johns Hopkins Hospital," "The Fire Music," (*U of Pitt Press*, 1986); "In the End We Are All Light," *The New Yorker*; **Kelly Seiver**— "One Life," *The Oregonian*, Sunday poetry column; **Allison Smythe**— "The Way a Day Can Break," *Relief Journal*; **Thom Tammaro**, "A Dream of My Father," *Indiana Imprint*; **Patricia Wellingham-Jones**— "The Flow," *Don't Turn Away: Poems about breast cancer*, and *Song of the San Joaquin Journal* (reprinted); "Don't Turn Away," *Lummox Journal, Don't Turn Away: Poems about Breast Cancer*," (PWJ Publishing, 2000); "Suppose the Owl Calls My Name," *bovine free Wyoming*; "Pictures for an Artist," *Atlantic Breast Cancer Net* (Canada), *Inglis House Poetry*

Workshop Contest; "Walk of the One-Breasted Women," *EDGZ*; **Martin Willitts, Jr.**— "The Hospital Approaches as a Prescription for Pain," *5th Gear*; "Letter from Karen" and "Captive", *hotmetalpress. net*; all three reprinted in *Lowering the Nets of Light* (*Pudding House Publications*, 2007); **Alessio Zanelli** — "Mr Palmer," *Poetry Monthly,* UK, and reprinted in *Straigth Astray* (Troubator, UK, 2005).

Table of Contents:

9

Foreword

January 2006, Frances Willitts was diagnosed with lung cancer. She had been a breast cancer survivor for more than twenty years. The cancer had been detected early and she was placed on chemo. Her body began to reject the chemo; she contacted pneumonia; and died in August 2006. I started writing poems about her death as a way to deal with my loss and along the way I began to share these poems with other people who had experiences with cancer. They started talking about how the poems made them feel better and helped them to deal with their own experiences. They started sending me poems about cancer. This gave me the idea of sharing therapeutic writing with others.

This was a grant-funded project that focused on an innovative approach to therapeutic poetry which I hoped will be beneficial for cancer patients, cancer survivors, and those who are close to them as they deal with issues of despair, love, loss, grief, and hope. The initial target was the public in Broome and Chenango County in New York; but it also included many other writers. We had a writer's workshop beginning with a memoir and then we edited it to a free verse poem. This anthology is the second part of the grant and it contains many of the writers from the workshop or the two counties. The next part is a poetry reading from this book.

According to The American Cancer Society (www.cancer.org), there are 100 different types of cancer: 559, 550 people died from cancer in the United States; 40,460 from breast cancer; 52,180 from leukemia; 160,390 from lung cancer; and 27,050 from prostate cancer.

I lost my father and wife to cancer. My brother, sister, and mother all had cancer. I have annual cancer checkups. How about you? I want to live to see my new grandson graduate from high school. I hope you find a reason to fight cancer. I recommend that you visit the Internet website, www.acscn.org for the American Cancer Society Network. If you want to continue to write and possibly publish more poems about cancer please contact www.survivorsreview.org.

I want to express thanks the Chenango County Council of the Arts and its board for choosing this project as the only project in 2007. I want to praise Deb Whitman for her advice on the grant proposal. I want to express gratitude to Linda S. Lewis-Moors for her support and connections with the American Cancer Society, the American Heart Association, and the Chenango County Memorial Hospital and its health network which all contributed to this project. Carolina Sineni shared poems about our loved ones and helped focus my drive to make this project a reality. Finally, I want to thank all the writers who participated in this project and contributed to make this into such a wonderful, heart-felt anthology.

Kathy Abrahams
Empty

Blue mood descends,
Feeling bereft,
Images of slashing knives.
Stripped of womanhood's
      Fruit bowl

    Hysterectomy.

Kathy Abrahams, Western Australia. Her work has been published in
*FreeXpresSion, Centoria Poetry Journal, Lucidity, The Mozzie, Micropress, Readers'
World, Vermont Ink, Realeight Ezine, The Dawn,* and *The Australian Writers' Journal.*

"I had a hysterectomy in September last year, after it was found that my womb
was in a pre-cancerous state."

Christine Orchanian Adler
Unearthed

For Sarah Adler

As a girl, you used to paint
low on the walls in the corner of your room,
tiny trees and flowers, undetected.

Soon boarding school called;
I was left to rearrange
the furniture, unearth your garden. We spoke

later; you laughed at the standoffs
that brought on those small
rebellions. Such colorful pictures,

defiantly raised your young
psyche then. Yet you haven't outgrown
the consolation of such things:

now eighteen, home from school,
I hear you slip nights
into the bathroom—the one I can't bear

to enter for the mess—and crouch
on the floor in the corner. Now
instead of creating, you peel

the paper. Flowers fall off
in little strips leaving, beneath,
bare blue walls.

I knew my body would
betray me as I aged, yet death
is not the mid-life crisis I'd expected.

But what I'm most sorry for
is what my illness does to us:
strips me by layers of physical strength,

peels you slowly in little
emotional strips until
all that's left is bare and blue.

Yet you are the unlucky one:
soon my aching will end.
But you will remain and be forced

to rearrange, unable to speak
with me about whatever you may
happen to suddenly unearth.

Christine Orchanian Adler, Yorktown Heights, NY. Her poetry has appeared in *The Furnace Review*, *Penumbra*, *LiteraryMama.com*, and *Coal: A Poetry Anthology*. Holding a Master of Arts degree in Creative Writing from Manhattanville College, she is Editorial Consultant of the literary journal, *Inkwell*, and Editor of Westchester *Parent* magazine.

"My poem is written for my sister-in-law and her family, all of whom were affected by her cancer."

Timor Avitzour

I could have been now
A tranquil girl, with a smile on her face,
And not perpetually cross.
A serene and confident girl,
Who doesn't fear every shadow.
I could have been now
A regular schoolgirl,
And a girl who returns home from school
With quick, light steps,
Without arriving panting and in pain.
I could have
Joined all the trips and camps
That I missed and will go on missing.
Slept at night, with pleasant dreams,
Made peace with myself — no one's perfect.
I could have
Had friends
Who come to my home and host me at theirs,
And all could have been self-evident,
And clear, that I truly deserve this.
I could have had something to do with my life,
Accept love from my sisters
And finally stop weeping
And be fourteen and five months old.
I could
Have
Been.

Timor Avitzour, Jerusalem, Israel, (translated by her mother, Susan Avitzour). "These are translations of poems written in Hebrew by my daughter, Timora, who died of leukemia at the age of eighteen, on January 5, 2001."

"'I could have been now' was written during her three-year remission. The other poem was written after the cancer returned."

Timor Avitzour

It
is
spreading further and further
and
conquering every spot that had been free
Poisonous, black malicious
Chuckling of devastation, of evil, of defenselessness, of some
dark power
Extending long and emaciated and terrible and destructive arms
that grow
like some horrible nightmare from which we've not awakened and
we'll not awaken
ever
And twist and twi-
st
and distort
and deform
and hold on

Hold fast by the nails
Hold and do not let go
Hold fast and wound
And if it does not bring death
it will bring destruction of some other kind
Because there are no few kinds
(to each his own destruction)
Here it's
bringing

Carol Willette Bachofner
Carol's Breast

My friend Carol has lost a breast. I imagine
her searching for it everywhere, bright visions
of this lost part of herself filling up her days.
She puts up notices, sends out flyers, offers
a reward. The aching on her chest, the space
beneath her nightgown, rudely reminds her
that this is a loss where no seeking, no money
offered, no begging will serve to act as remedy.
She must grieve the lost part and survive it.

Thousands of women are her sisters with losses
like hers beneath silk blouses. We pass daily
in traffic, on sidewalks, in hallways. In our full days,
theirs have empty spaces we can not know. We do not
see the purple lines where surgeons opened them. We
can not feel their fear. Wingless birds can no longer soar;
and these breastless ones flap in desperate imbalance,
trying to get relief from their own gravity. We do not see
them struggle or offer to help. We are afraid of them.

My friend's breast is not really lost; she gave it up
to save herself, to save a life with her family, to spend
nights safe in her husband's arms. I sometimes wonder
if her husband bears hatred towards the gone breast for
trying to take her from him. Does he lay his hand over
the emptiness and remember the lushness of her, the sweet
milky taste of her on his tongue? Do her daughters watch in
fear by their mirrors, looking for doom on their chests?
I look at my own two breasts, safe and round, and I feel guilty.

Carol Willette Bachofner, Rockland, Maine. Her work has been published in *Prairie Schooner*, *The Cream City Review*, *The Comstock Review*, *The Mochila Review*, *Pebble Lake*, and others. Her chapbook, *Daughter of the Ardennes Forest*, was published (Main Street Rag, 2007). She holds an MFA in Writing (Poetry) from Vermont College and is founding editor of *Pulse*, an online literary journal which can be found at www.heartsoundpress.com.

"'Carol's Breast' is about my friend, who indeed has survived breast cancer, having had a mastectomy. [She also survived kidney cancer.] She and her husband are a very close couple and the cancer seems only to have made them closer. Her husband (Jim) is a childhood friend of my husband."

Barbara Joan Tiger Bass

Hospitalization

the gown
blue snow-flake print
white tie-ups
says NEVER TO LEAVE HOSPITAL

so many tubes run into
the veins of my lover
his hugs tentative reminders
a body I sweated with

dry now and thinner
he holds up the plastic lines
as if to allow passage
slings them over his shoulder

pushes his I.V. pole
down the corridor

Barbara Joan Tiger Bass, Oakland, CA, coaches writers and teaches Creative Writing workshops through her business, Enjoy Learning. Her poetry has been published in *VeRT*, *Peralta Press*, *Literary Mama*, and her musical theater piece, *Koc(h)ka*, was produced and performed in Sacramento, Ca. in 2006.

"My poem was written while my late husband, Larry Lajmer (1953-2000) was suffering with cancer. I was his primary caregiver. I hope my poem will offer some comfort to others."

Shaindel Beers
Surgery

Cold seeps
up   through the thin mat
they've rolled me onto
settles   in my pelvic bones
        Second time
under
the knife   in four weeks
First time
to see   why the bleeding
hasn't stopped for months
Second time
removing cells threatening
to turn into cancer
        Each time a microscopic
unsexing   more bits / more chunks / of me
removed
Next time (if there is one)   I will
        float   up
        listen in as they work   find out
if the small-talk jokes they make   as their faces
        become   blurry   are for them
or for me
If I really look ten years younger
        than my chart says   If the reason
they are sparing my uterus   is so I can have
        a little girl with stoic grey eyes
gold sunflowers   in their centers

Shaindel Beers, Pendleton. OR, is currently a professor of English at Blue
Mountain Community College in Pendleton, Oregon. Her poetry, fiction, and
social commentary have appeared in *Willow Review*, *Poetry Miscellany*, *Hunger
Mountain*, and numerous other journals and publications. She serves as Poetry
Editor of *Contrary* www.contrarymagazine.com.

"I am not a cancer survivor, technically, but I have had medical procedures done
to prevent cancer. I have lost friends to cancer and have seen friends survive."

Sally Bellerose
Bye Bye Barbara

She went slowly,
with very little meat
between the skin
and spine.

Still,
until the end
　　　she tried
to make a straight line
　　　of bone.

Hungry all the time.

The big surprise was her eyes,
how they bulged
with the world
getting bigger in her orbits
as she died.

Sally Bellerose, Northampton MA, has won grants and fellowships including an NEA, The Barbara Deming Fiction Prize, and The Rick DeMartinis Award. Her recently published work can be read in current issues of *Rock and Sling*, *The Binnacle*, *The Journal of Humanistic Anthropology*, *The Boston Literary Magazine*, *Passenger*, *Cutthroat*, *Saint Ann's Review*, and *Cup of Comfort for Writers*. The first Chapter of her novel, *The GirlsClub* appears on www.SallyBellerose.com.

"'Bye Bye Barbara' was written 15 years ago for a friend who died of lung cancer."

Richard Bernstein
Some Guys

1.

And so this evening we enter, all trial and error,
half ageless, half passing,
our path hardening through a smother of hemlock,
brush of pine, the ironing in
and out of mystery.
A few under the hoist of aluminum canoes,
a few fraying like dusk through brittle leaves
along seams of half-drunk October geese, a few
who would rather starve in the avalanche of all-at-once
than endure the gradual hunger for the years,
a few who are hungry and happy for the hunger.

Somewhere in the forest are fish. We believe this
regardless of whether or not it's true.
In my pack is a bottle of water, a turkey sandwich
on whole grain, an extra pair of socks,
some hooks and worms, my father's ashes.
Each of us has his own. We also have a tent.

2.

October is an empty room, full of everything we know.
Her face is young, blushed where the surface fades.
Her hair shines. Beneath the veil of fruit
she carries the scent of her birth. From a distance
she has the look of someone who could be loved.
She's lived in the forest a long time,
reminds me of someone I might have known.
I lean into her, put my head on her lap,
breathe when she breathes
the absence of absolute night in the improbable sky.
It might as well be 2:00 a.m. on 8th Avenue , or a dream
that is not yet a dream or anything other than what it is.
See, she's already begun to change.

3.

Even when they cleared away the brush, filled the putrid marsh
where my father's kidney had been, and part of his lung
gave him space enough to build
twelve years with a clear view of the uncertain horizon;
even when he sat in the kitchen for hours on a spackle can
as the light from his cigarette drifted into a magazine print
of "The Oxbow" on an otherwise frameless wall,
or listened to the scratch of Smetana's "Moldau"
on the old phonograph; only the crab cherry,
pressed against his bedroom window,
weeped and only sometimes in early fall,
in the evening, an hour or two after the coffee had cooled.

4.

I won't presume to tell you how little the forest feels,
or how much, how we could scatter the dead a hundred times,
a thousand, and would, and still not get it right, or wrong.
What I will say is this: Somewhere in the forest
is a fish. Whether there is or isn't
doesn't seem to make much difference.

Richard Bernstein, Norwich , NY, has a M.A. in English from Binghamton
University , Binghamton , New York . He has been an English teacher for 21 years
at the Norwich High School where he has led the high school poetry team to
statewide championship for 7 years. He is adjunct professor of English at (SUNY)
Morrisville State College. He has poems published in the *Georgia Review*

Gary Blankenship
Poetic States VII — Delaware

Caesar Rodney
rode through the July night, thunder
and storm his sole companions,
to cast a vote to break a deadlock
that allowed Jefferson's Declaration.

"The oddest looking man in the world,"*
his face marred with painful cancer,
he did not live to see the Constitution
his home state was first to ratify.

Flip a Delaware quarter on its back
and see sick Caesar's heroic ride.
Paul Revere may have warned the farms
the British were on the march,

but Delaware's Rodney rode his black horse
as hard for the colony's independence
against his friends' and neighbors' wishes.

*John Adams

Gary Blankenship, Bremerton, WA, is a retired manager who dabbles in poetry and publishing. He is CEO of Santiam Publishing and published the online journals, *MindFire Renewed* and *FireWeed*, both at www.mindfirerenew.com. Gary has been published on the web and in a variety of paper publications. His volume of poetry, *River Transformed* is available at people.lulu.com/users.

"Caesar Rodney is one of our genuine heroes and as far as I know one of the few with cancer."

Sydney H. Brisker
Cremation

The beautiful face,
the perfect nose,
the smile that melted my heart.
Up in smoke.

The bosom on which
I laid my head
for comfort at end of day.
Up in smoke.

The firm white thighs
that cradled the mound of Venus
where I left the essence of life,
Up in smoke.

The long, slim legs
that encircled my body
during the dance of love.
Up in smoke.

The love in my heart
that sustained me all those years,
stays with me, and did not go
Up in smoke.

Sydney H. Brisker, Los Angeles, CA, is a retired architect who has been writing poetry, short stories and essays since 1938. He was co-editor of *The Architecture of Ricordo Legorreta.* His experience as a WW II Navy Lieutenant in the anthology *Very Truly Ours, Letters from America's fighting Men; Grace under Fire: Letters of Faith in Times of War*; and, *War Letters: Extraordinary Correspondence from American Wars.* His recent poem appeared in *Eclipse.*

In 1993, after 51 years of marriage his wife died of ovarian cancer.

Angie Chuang
When I Will Know

Is there an arm that I have to take this on? His voice grows soft
around the edges. His thick hands seem to hold the Velcro jaws of
the blood-pressure cuff at bay. After my automatic no, puzzled, he
looks at me, skeptical. Are you sure? he asks. Lymphedema, of course
— he thinks I'm a breast cancer patient. The oncology department's
a guessing game, a test of medical probability. I assumed the white-
haired man outside was prostate; the teenager in a wheelchair and
a knit cap over her smooth scalp, leukemia. And me? Thirty-three,
female, healthy-looking — breast cancer was a good guess. But no,
I want to say, I've always been a little different. Mature for my age.
I had a tumor more in vogue among 60-year-olds. You don't need to
worry about my arm, but I am thinking about the scar that smiles
across my lower abdomen, still feisty and red. I say nothing and
offer him my right arm. I'm going to have to hold your arm, he says,
cradling it gently, so gently, and wrapping his meaty thumb around
the crook of my elbow. He still suspects I have lymphedema. I
study his weighty silver watch, hanging off his downy wrist, marking
seconds into the linoleum. I imagine him letting go, and what
happens next: The rrrrip of the cuff coming off, the scratch of the
pen as he jots down 122 over 65 on the clipboard, the silence as I
wait for Dr. Lehman, the whoosh of the hydraulic door as he strides
in and I study his placid, horse-like face for a sign.

Angie Chuang, Portland, OR, is a journalist in who writes poetry and literary
non-fiction about the intersections of cultures, or as Salman Rushdie describes,
"world's in collision." Her poetry has been published in CALYX, *Mizna, The
Grove Review, Windfall: A Journal of Poetry of Place* and other journals and
anthologies. She received a 2007 Oregon Literary Fellowship in Creative Non-
Fiction for a memoir centered on a 2004 trip to Afghanistan. An excerpt of
that memoir appears in the *Lonely Planet's* travel-writing anthology, *Tales from
Nowhere.*

She is an ovarian cancer survivor.

Maggie Creshkoff
Why Losing a Job Seems So Unimportant Now

On Sunday, all her words came slow
And pale and weak from spitting blood
The chemo kills her faster than the cancer ever did.

Her face is old, all skin, all bones
Her body's like a starving child's,
A belly swollen full with no new life for her

Twelve years ago they found that lump,
They took her breasts, they burned her bones
A dozen years of hope and poisoned pills

and all for this:

to feel the wind through hair as thin as thread
to see the sun through leaves of newest green
to hear the birds call through the slender trees
to touch her mother's face despite the dark.

Maggie Creshkoff, Port Deposit, MD, is a potter and a poet who lives on a farm in rural Maryland with far too many cats. She won 1st and 2nd prize in the Queen Anne's County Contest in 2005, a 3rd prize in 2004 (publication in *Delmarva Monthly*). She has had articles published in *Ceramics Monthly, Studio Potter, Mason Dixon Arrive*, as well as in our local paper, the *Cecil Whig*. "Our poetry group, *Lunchlines* (the same group that Peter Goodwin belongs to) publishes a chapbook every other year.

"My friend Mary Anne Ragan has breast cancer for 12 years, which has metastasized to the bones. She can no longer undergo chemotherapy, they're all killing her. She is a few years younger than I, she's not quite 50. She lives in a house set high in tall trees, loves birds and wild plants, and makes intricate amulets from beads and wire. I remember to the day when she told me of the diagnosis, how unreal it all seemed, as full of life as she was. And now she's emptying out, bit by bit. It is so damn unfair. I'm not the one to say, but it doesn't seem as if she's had that much of a life."

Patrick Dacey
Eulogy for My Mother: January 15th, 2003

In our house, an angel painted the rooms
danced through the hallways
and laughed; she had a beautiful laugh.

There were no doors closed in our house,
you could come right in,
and wherever she was
her heart was ready to heal your own.

She lived like you or I,
except her own self was much less important.
When someone felt defeated, when someone
wanted that defeat,
she took it on, she showed them what it meant to fight,
she gave them hope.
And the people who confided in her,
the angel stayed with them too.

It was the three of us in the house,
and together we grew,
saw each other change,
gave each other love and support and guidance
and whenever we left for places unknown
the three of us went together.

I have learned through her that there's no greater trust
than the one given when love is uncontrollable.
To have faith in this is to live the way my mother did
She loved us all

With the kindness she gave from her heart,
and the beauty she gave to our lives: a mother, a daughter,
a friend and an angel has flown from that world
but remains in this.

Patrick Dacey, Syracuse, NY, has a MFA fellowship at Syracuse University, has publications in *The Smithsonian Magazine*, *Fiction Attic*, and *Bridges: A journal of multicultural writing*.

"My mother passed away four years ago from ovarian cancer after battling for three years. She underwent four treatments of chemotherapy. The fourth was the most successful, however the harshest and caused an allergic reaction inside her, which stopped blood flow to the brain one day. She continued to live, but barely, and passed away three weeks later. Cancer has had a long history in our family; both of my grandfathers died of cancer as well."

Barbara Daniels
The Cancer Patient Addresses Her Husband

There are holes in beauty, hollows
in birds' bones, light years between the stars.

Elegant, undulant fog drifts and sighs.
Or is it trees sighing, oaks dangling scalloped leaves

that cling through winter storms?
Crows ready themselves to row once more

over emptiness. I walk again, working against
the ache of it. You know the neighbors watch

my daily laboring. Always some joy—
yelow striped head of a kinglet, robins flocked

where snow opens under pines.
I pull fresh bread from the oven.

Yeasty smell in the warmth all day.
Comfort me with peaches, with hot broth.

And what? The old ways of touching?
It's lovely to lie down together,

you beside my bare body. What
are we made of? You kiss my breasts

and bald head. Fierce kisses, bright
red scars. I believe I am not yet dying.

Barbara Daniels
Periwinkle

My big book of cancer
lists 68 words for pain.
I light two candles, eat saltines

and start the OxyContin.
Move a button from bowl to bowl
each time I drink eight ounces of water.

It's a brave world, wan leaves
in the new snow on the hill.
An enormous sky.

I spend the day watching the light.
At dawn there's a half hour of rose
through ice at the roofline.

By five at night the green
of the pines deepens to black.
The snow and the sky turn

the same blue white.
What's that blue my mother likes?
Periwinkle?

Named for the funneled flower.
Blue scatters into the night,
petalled shadows.

I tie a blue bandana
over my bald head. Chill filters in.
I move the flowers my mother sent

so I can see them when I look up
from my heavy book. Each is still
perfect, ice blue and tender.

Barbara Daniels
Begging

> I beg my bones to be good.
>   Lucille Clifton

I beg my pulse,
                my fecal smear
on a doctor's test kit,
my blood in marked vials.

Come right this time.

Bones, lattice me, my pruned self
hung on you,
greedy, striving.

Stay warm, blue heart.
Stop kicking and bawling.

Help me, apple.
Carry me
   on your smooth round back.

Barbara Daniels, Sicklerville, NJ. Her book, *Rose Fever*, will be published by WordTech Press in 2008. She received two Individual Artist Fellowships from the New Jersey State Council on the Arts, earned an MFA in poetry at Vermont College, and teaches at Camden County College in New Jersey. Her chapbook, *The Woman Who Tries to Believe*, won the Quentin R. Howard Prize. Her poems have appeared in *The Louisville Review*, *Natural Bridge*, *Blueline*, and others.

"I'm a survivor of ovarian cancer."

Susan Deer Cloud
Hoop Dream

A few in our family fought against cremation.
But you wanted your cancer-bitten body burnt
when you left here. I saw how it was with you
in those last days before you moaned
into your coma, eyes half open
until you died. The doctor
arrived, coaxed them shut at last.
I saw how the pain stole all
belief from you.

What I want is to be able
to say something about that year,
the kind of seemingly wise words
that land people on talk shows.
But I have no Oprah wisdom to give —
except I don't get TV anymore
and smile out windows
at the birds I feed.

The cancer took a breast, pecked
at your liver, snapped your neck.
You died in winter and we waited
until May to drive your ashes up
to the mountain where our father's
war-shot body lay. We scattered you,
tried not to fall sobbing to our knees as we
let drop from our doubled over hands
your high cheek-boned face, cat-like
frame, rain-grey eyes flowered
with shattered fire.

What is there to say
when a mother dies that way?
Why so much cancer? That we did cry,

careful not to look at or hear each other?
And a rainbow appeared around the sun.
We watched it sideways, until my sister decided,
"That's Mom saying she's still with us."
We left your ashes behind with Dad, dreaming
you were lovers again in some "next world."
In town, the hoop circling the sun was gone.

Susan Deer Cloud, Binghamton, NY: Susan Deer Cloud (Blackfoot, Mohawk, Seneca,) has poems and stories published in numerous journals & anthologies. Her latest book is *The Last Ceremony* (Foothills Press). She has received various awards and fellowships, including a New York State Foundation for the Arts Fellowship, a Chenango County Council for the Arts Individual Artist Grant and a National Endowment for the Arts Literature Fellowship in Poetry.

"'My 53rd Birthday' is a poem I wrote about my grandmother. She died of brain cancer. 'Hoop Dream' refers to my maternal grandmother and her death from brain cancer."

Susan Deer Cloud
My 53rd Birthday

Another birthday, my 53rd. But that doesn't satisfy me.
I prefer to say I'm really old, ancient as stars.
Sometimes I have felt that oldness in this strange
autumn when the leaves waited so long to turn, and then
only into muted fires. Warmest September on record.
But the wooly bear caterpillars crawling across roads
have black bands so long the brown hardly shows.
I pick them up in my hands, feel delicate hairs
on my heart lines, pray they're wrong about the harsh
winter to come. Sometimes I see my grandmother.
Always the same image — me walking up School Street
to meet her around the time I knew she'd be walking home
from work at Dratty's Bed and Breakfast, same age
I am now. My grandfather had already died of his heart attack.
She didn't know she had brain cancer, yet. Widowhood
forced her to rent out her house, move in with us. I knew
she was poor, but only now after my divorce at absolute mid-life
do I understand just how poor, scared, she must have been.
So I keep holding the wooly bears in my hands —
walk up the street, skipping when I glimpse my grandmother
in her green flowered dress and auburn hair softened
into hints of flame, the way the trees are this year.
Finally, I reach her. I show her the caterpillars that appear
never to turn into butterflies. I set them down on Catskill lawn,
take my grandmother's hand. We never speak in this memory —
a sepia photograph in an oval frame. We just walk to
my parents' house, feeling each other's hands like small wings
beating against heartbreak. Lately my bones hurt far inside.
Mornings my feet ache so I worry I will fall down the stairs,
until my Persian cat dashes to greet me. Her exuberance
stops me from falling. I hope I was like that for my grandmother
when my exuberance led me up School Street. I wonder
if I, too, will die when I'm not quite 60. I wish I knew.
I'd like to take a plane back to Paris or fly somewhere
utterly new, maybe a patch of unfound land

in the Amazon. Or maybe I'd find the family castle in England
my grandmother told me about, and I'd be Queen for a Day
and banish poverty, fear, loneliness, and death. Yes, I'm old
as the stars going on 53 and wondering for the zillionth time
what I am doing here, what we are for, what our love means
when our hearts break into ash, our ash rots in the ground.
I keep walking up School Street, greeting my grandmother.
I am smiling at her. I am grabbing the hand of my future.
I am going home.

Lorene Delany-Ullman
The Radiation Diaries

I.   The Salton Sea

Impoverished trough of salt,
an ancient lake is renewed
by the floodwaters of the Colorado.

To prevent goiters (hard g
similar to geiger and God)
salt is impregnated with iodine.

As a child, I floated in saltwater
so thick it formed a crust,
a crystalline imprint of

the Salton Sea; my belly turned
upward to unnerve the sky.
Where the brine wells were once
tapped for salt, now lies a popular resort.

II.   The Cliché of Hands

The shadows are consumed by the hand, even the sunlight concedes
to the whiteness of her hand; assume a woman walking with a man.
Her fingers hinged to his mid-spine as if to close in the blackness
of his suit; her palm cupped to hold in the remnants of intimacy
thinking of escape.

*

Before rush hour traffic, I drive into the morning fog and cannot
separate memory from imagination. Still, what is invisible to our
eyes can be measured. Out of the fog, a flurry of translucent images,
until one is caught in the chrome of the side-view mirror: plastic
gloves from a nearby-toppled truck; the hands amiss.

III.   3 Feet

Isola-
(shun), the dis
stance is 3

feet for Safe-
Tee. I am
radio—

active. Glo
girl wants to
swallow three

IV.   To Madame Curie

When your mind is quiet
is when you are most afraid.

Sleep is never your friend
until you discover that

you own an opaque body.
Anemia and bone

pain are the side-effects.
When will I know my own body?

I hear you say: trust the dream
and an unexpected discovery occurs.

V.   The Half-life of an Isotope

The half-life of an isotope is longer
than it took for God to create the world.

Even the doctor makes the sign of the cross
in mockery of the monster I have become.

I swallowed a miniature Chernobyl.
My body is both the shelter

of myself (from myself) and the fallout.
Isolation is the white coat with no hands;

the hospital door closed
as if isotopes can't penetrate wood.

VI.   Entities that are Synthetic

Fuels, fibers, and pharmaceuticals.
Man-made, no hand-made,
made by hand, not a man's hand,
but a woman's hand, our hands that make
us man not animal—derivatives of man
are not equal to woman, origins of manual, or
the root of artisan. This dexterity leads to artifice
or craft-brother, but not right-handedness.

VII.   The Impurities of the Parable

The construct of impurity is as ancient as the "tell" or the
archaeological mound that holds history buried and untouched.
(Each telling of the parable is another hillock). Desirous or not,
contamination holds within itself: infect, impure, corrupt. Here,
the impurities remain unnamed: an American woman, fair and
freckled, nondescript of dress and religion seeks the hand (four
fingers & thumb, nails clean, some calluses acceptable) of her
husband, the man who stands three feet from her door.

Lorene Delany-Ullman, Irvine, CA, received her MFA from the University of
California, Irvine in June 2003. She has been published in *Elixir, Crab Creek
Review, Washington Square, Identitytheory, Perihelion, Vermillion Literary Project,
Seastories.org, Versal* and *Upstreet*. She was the managing editor for *Faultline*, UC
Irvine's literary journal. She teaches composition and poetry at UC Irvine. She
is one of the founding members of the *Casa Romantica Poetry Reading Series*, a
committee of local southern California writers who sponsor and organize monthly
poetry readings in south Orange County.

"I am a survivor of thyroid cancer."

Liz Dolan
What I Did Not Say

From the steps of her house,
late afternoon light candling her hair,
my sister and I overlook Cupsaw Lake
where her six children swam
and flourished like local fauna.
She tells me to tell her husband
the house looks great. He wants to sell,
too much work, wants to tee off in Florida.
Before I leave, she tells me she speaks everyday
to John, a friend, who died last year.
She laughs, I'll be joining him soon.
Rushing, I check my bag for my keys,
my wallet, my makeup case,
give her a hug and am stung
by her bones protruding like nettles.
Good days, bad days, she says.
I look at her. I did not want to hear
what I did not say.

Liz Dolan, Rehoboth Beach, DE, is a former English teacher and administrator. She is most proud of the alternative school she ran in the Bronx and her eight grandchildren. She has published poems, memoirs and short stories in *Philadelphia Stories, New Delta Review, Rattle, Natural Bridge, Illuminations, Mudlark, Bardsong, Windhover* and other journals. A 2005 Pushcart Prize nominee in fiction and 2006 nominee in poetry, she was recently a finalist in The Dogfish Head chapbook contest. She received honorable mention for best poem of the year in *Gin Bender Literary Review*, and third in the *Pure Sea Glass* poetry contest. She has been selected as associate artist in residence with poet Sharon Olds. She received an emerging professional fellowship in poetry from the DDOA. She is on the poetry board of *Philadelphia Stories*.

"I am writing about loved ones who have had cancer; two have died."

Joseph A. Farina
Pink Ribbons

she took my hand
and spoke to me of lumps
nesting in her breast-
i held her in her trembling-
she held me in my fear-
both of us afflicted -
the shadow of winter in our eyes

Joseph A. Farina, Sarnia ON, Canada: Joseph A. Farina practices Law in Canada. He won second prize in the *Sarnia Observer* "My Hometown" contest for his essay "My New Home Town." His poems have been published in *Green's Magazine, Quills Canadian Poetry Magazine, Ascent, The Tower Poetry Magazine, Pyramid Magazine, Memoirs, Sweet Lemons* (anthology), *Writings with a Sicilian Accent,* and *Witness* (anthology).

"In the space of a few weeks my good friend Rodney and my son were diagnosed with Cancer. My son survived: my friend did not. The ordeal caused both them and myself distress, and gave birth to a collection of poems *The Cancer Chronicles: a parent's journey,* Serengeti Press. All royalties go to the Cancer Society of Canada."

Peter D Goodwin
CANCER (An Unfinished Poem)

Stage 1

She celebrates
her comfortable retirement
her pleasures
and her good health.
Cancer smiles.

She looks after her body
exercises
eats wisely
fells good.
So does Cancer.

I look after you
she told her body;
you look after me.
Cancer stretches.

All her life she worked hard.
All her life she struggled
against the jerks, the boors and the frauds
against self serving bureaucrats
and other back stabbers.
All her life she triumphed
even when she did not win
she triumphed.
She refused to be a victim.
She had never met Cancer.

On a beautiful day
enjoying her morning coffee
she paid no attention

when she burped.
Cancer knocked

Stage 2

Like the Mongolian Horde of old
Cancer has a secret weapon
the breadth of fear
the hushed whispers
the word
just the word
cancer.

Cancer whispers cancer.
Abandon all hope
Ima goin' to get you
accept your fate.

Cancer is busy
collecting its clients
filling the clinics
a callous calculation
of a business of growth
Cancer grows
business grows
and many have work
a diabolical calculation.
Soon those who work with Cancer
will never leave
caught within Cancer' s
fatal embrace.

Cancer is tough
a real HE man
throw it a punch

HE bounces back
smiling
Come on
make my day
I eat this stuff.

Cancer plays hide and seek:
see me — I'm gone
Find me — I'm elsewhere
Cut me — I'm off
Remove me — I'll be back
Ignore me — I'm waiting for you
Kill me — forgetaboutit.

Will you dance with me? Cancer asks.
You will dance! Cancer repeats.
Dance the jet, dance the hop
Hear the music
Dance the flow, dance the flop
Dance the disco with me
around and around we go
Listen to the beat
follow the beat
my beat
Around and around we go
around and around we go.
Until I let go.
I never let go.

Stage 3

Cancer sleeps, smiling
snoring content
others listen and wait.

Health returns.

Normal life returns.
Visits to the doctor routine
a boring break.
Life is good.
Cancer pounces.

Flirtation is over
Now we embrace
in a dance for life
until one falls from exhaustion.
Cancer feels fit.

Don't be angry, Cancer smiles.
Are you angry with the weather?
The movements of the moon?
The tides?
I am the weather and the tides.
Your weather
Just like life—
and death

Peter D Goodwin, North East, MD. "I am continually amazed at the courage and dedication of so many people who stay within the cancer networks, helping other people cope with these terrible diseases. So I tip my hat to you — that you are willing to put so much work into this project which must be very painful."

"My wife has been struggling against (kidney) cancer for five years, so far successfully. We know how it will end but not when. I have been working on this poem for several years, usually in waiting rooms, a word or a line here, or a stanza there, so it has grown, like the medical files or the tumors. I hope it will be many, many years before this poem is finished. My wife is alive today only because of all our modern technology, but the hospitals are strange, impersonal places."

Tzivia Gover
July Fifteenth

Cindy returned to work today,
her dress, the color of peaches,
her new wig soft, as a doll's hair,
her left arm bruised from the IV.
Before, every hospital stay had been a battle won.
Today she said, "I don't want to go back there again."
She made "there" sound like more than just a building or a room.
She stood at my desk.
I ignored the instant message flashing on my screen,
and the whine of the copy machine.
She said she'd had a dream
that she was never coming back
to work and I
was sitting at her desk.
"I would never do that,"
I promised, grateful
for any true assurance
I could offer.

Tzivia Gover, Holyoke, MA. She is a writer and educator. Her poems have been published in journals and anthologies including *The Bark*, *Lilith*, *The Berkshire Review* and dozens of others. She received my MFA in Creative Nonfiction from Columbia University. She currently teach poetry to teen mothers in a GED program in Holyoke, Mass.

"My poems were written in honor of my friend and co-worker, Cindy Klimoski, who died of cancer last year."

Adele C. Graghty
Death in 'C' Ward

 She waits for comets
bleeding fiery ash;
no ransom forthcoming,
drifting beneath

morphine cool sheets,
awaiting the next
pleasure push from
faceless angels. In the dark,

she's offering arms to an abyss
for syringe bites and cobra cuffs,
which meter her statistics
like the descent

of translucent feathers,
falling lighter and softer with
each breath, 'till like an egg,
slippery with mother ooze,

she pushes her calcified head
into the hereafter,
singeing wings in the birth canal
and is reborn, a believer.

Adele C. Graghty, Sheffield, South Yorkshire, United Kingdom. Born in New York and now residing in the United Kingdom, Adele C. Geraghty is a recipient of The US National Women's History Award for *Women's Related Poetry and Essay*. Her current work is *"Skywriting in the Minor Key: Women, Words, Wings."*

"Many of my poems are dedicated to my maternal grandmother who died of breast cancer."

Lois I. Greenberg
Chemo

"I don't want this to interfere with your life."
Reginald Pugh, MD

headband tourniquet
slows the flow of chemicals

to the brain
dams creative juices

poets drown in bubbles
on a downward drip

the smell of antiseptic
lingers long beyond this tick

ruins my appetite
for rhyme and meter

if you've been there
you know how clocks

chase minutes drag hours
I covet time never enough

sometimes too much
misery plods like a bad movie

in slow motion joy rushes by
on fast forward that hasty light

comes in handy in the dark
lethargy limits movement
I dance a slower step

Lois I. Greenberg, Pittsburgh, PA, a Licensed Clinical Social Worker, her work has appeared in *Paper Street*, *Pittsburgh Post-Gazette*, *HEArt* (Human Equity Through Art), the *National Book Foundation* anthology, *The Eternal Fire*, *hotmetalpress*, and *writersalliance*. She is a member of the Pittsburgh Poetry Exchange and Advisory Board of *Paper Street*.

"In 1981, I was diagnosed with metastatic breast cancer, had a year of weekly chemo and a course of radiation. In 1993 I was diagnosed with a second primary (in the other breast), treated with lumpectomy and radiation and in 1997 had a recurrence of the original cancer in my supraclavicular node (shoulder) for which I received radiation. I am currently cancer free. At the time of the original diagnosis, I had two adolescent children and, as a single parent, was most anxious about survival. They needed me and I had to live. There were no other options! I was working full- time in a most supportive environment and my lover/friends/ family provided enough nurturance to see me through the hard time. Postscript: the therapy ended when I had pulmonary emboli (sometimes chemo does that) and then cried for three months - all the tears that I held back during that awful year finally flowed over the dam. Others have told me they hear the despair/ disgust with treatment but that the last two lines suggest a determination to move on — 'I dance a slower step" but I'm still dancin'.'"

Angela Hailey-Gregory
Falling

She wonders if dying feels like fall—
A gradual fading of the light
Sweet and sad and dim.
She senses the gravity of the earth beneath her feet,
Pulling her to obligation and rectitude,
Her back is straight and her fingers slim.

She folds things into little squares and rectangles
And places them carefully in the suitcase,
Pausing over each one to confirm its value and usefulness.
The rippled glass distorts her face like waves in a lake,
Sorrow is well-deep where she stands and breath
can sometimes be difficult.
She glances up again at the shadowed world
framed in the window

And walks out into the night,
Forgetting her suitcase on the bed.

Angela Hailey-Gregory, Oxford, NY. She wrote a scholarly article for journal
Mississippi Quarterly, was accepted into Binghamton University's Graduate
English Department last year as a doctoral candidate, but had to defer because
of her diagnosis, is am looking forward to attending this fall, however. She have
an undergraduate degree in theater from Wesleyan University, and a Master's in
English from SUNY Cortland."

"I am 37 years-old with a husband and two young girls. I have no history of
cancer in my family, and I was 'perfectly healthy' when a random blood test led
my doctors to discover a rare and large tumor, which had infiltrated my liver.
I was sent to Mt. Sinai where it took two very skilled surgeons to remove the
tumor. Since then, I have undergone 6 months of radiation and chemotherapy. I
am doing very well; however, my condition (the disease in conjunction with my
age, history, etc.) is very rare, and, as a result, none of my doctors can give me a
prognosis of any certainty."

Laura Heidy-Halberstein
In Utero

benevolent garden
one foreign seed draws first breath
inhale — divide

three spores are scattered
six cells seek sanctuary
exhale — multiply

malignant conception
each silent new spawn mutates
inhale — exhale

Laura Heidy-Halberstein, Alexandria, Va. Her poetry has been published in *Raintown Review, Solares Hill, Pebble Lake Review, Yellow Bat Press, Contemporary Rhyme, Hypertexts, Poet's Corner, Susquennah Quarterly*. Her work has also appeared in the Canadian Anthology, *"Rhyme and Reason"* and has been featured on *Verse Daily*.

"My poem was written for a friend who was suffering from both breast and uterine cancers."

Maryanne Hannan

Change

For Joe (1947-1980)

Nothing will change, he says,
home from the hospital, one leg
gone. I'll still be your daddy,
showing off a little for his girls' sake—
how easy to wield these crutches—
I'm a natural; could have been born a tripod.
Ignores their new shyness. Hugs his wife.
Important, he tells her, to make the best
Of a bad situation. Sitting's hard,
hip, half his pelvis gone; joking
Now I really am half-assed.
Up and down, out of his chair,
kitchen, living room, bathroom, practicing
until Time, he says, to start living normal again.
Puts on his red flannel shirt, old jeans.
His daughters bring home friends,
laugh, play cards, just like before
and buoyed by hope, the uncommon success,
he walks them, leaving, to the front door,
down the step, onto the porch,
first time out since the hospital.
One arm raised high, goodbye,
the other holding tight the crutch, and—
Shit!—his old jeans, loose,
slide down the one-hipped torso,
so much change
heaped around his ankle.

Maryanne Hannan, Delmar, NY. A former teacher, she has published poems in *Carquinez Poetry Review, Hampden-Sydney Poetry Review, Pebble Lake Review. Poet Lore, Sport Literate, upstreet* and *Xavier Review*. Her interview with Pattiann Rogers was recently anthologized in *Earthlight: Spiritual Wisdom for an Ecological Age*. In writing, she has found a way to deal with lacrimae rerum, "the tears in things."

"My husband died of cancer."

Joy Harold Helsing
Mastectomy

Cancer, the Crab
grabs my breast, fastens tight,
starts to feed on me. I think
just one thing: Get it off!
Get it off!

Finally, they do.

Joy Harold Helsing, Magalia, CA. As a college undergraduate she won two top awards for poetry in the *Atlantic Monthly* student writing contests. Her work has appeared in journals and she has published three chapbooks and one book, *Confessions of the Hare* (PWJ publishing).

"In 1993 I was diagnosed with inflammatory breast cancer and was treated with chemotherapy, modified radical mastectomy, radiation, and five years on tamoxifen. Although I still have some trouble with lymphedema, I did survive and have had no recurrence. I'm one of the lucky ones."

Joy Harold Helsing
The Knife

Five years ago a surgeon's knife
severed a breast
to save my life.

It was a fair exchange.
I still survive.
And I no longer need that chunk of flesh
to feed a child
or lure a lover.

But I have become a voyeur.
In spite of myself, I often stare
at high, firm mounds under tight clothing,
bare bosoms over daring décolletage,
bold bulges enhanced by clever brassieres.

I try not to be envious.
I have had my day.
Yet I can't stop feeling
such things should come in pairs,
not a lopsided solo
like mine.

And I want to warn
the beautiful, innocent girls
flaunting their beautiful, innocent wares —
enjoy it —
enjoy it
while you can.

Joy Harold Helsing
years after

mastectomy
she still dreams she has
both

and they are beautiful

William Heyen
Matrix

When I was a boy,
I found a mutilated turtle
emerging from mud.
Something, when it was young,
had broken its shell
almost in half,
but the shell,
as though welded with glossy solder,
had mended;
something had chewed
its back legs to the joints,
but its stumps were hard.
How did you survive,
I asked it,
But it was mute, still half adream
from its winter sleep.
I spoke to it,
warmed it in my boy's hands,
but it boxed itself up…..

For some time
after her mastectomy,
weeks of hospital and chemotherapy,
my wife woke towards me
in slow spirals,
as though from ether,
unsure of where we were
and how we'd live
in our new matrix
of scar and fear.
But it was April, again.
In windows before us,
as we changed her dressings,
the days rained, and warmed.

One morning, I pressed my lips
to her chest until, at last,
she believed,
and opened up to me.
Our answers so slow to come
that came.

William Heyen, Brockport, NY. His undergraduate degree is from State
University of New York at Brockport, where he is a professor of English and poet
in residence. H

William Heyen
Strawberries

My favorite slide of my wife before
our marriage during a moment of summer

she's perched on a picnic table her feet
on a bench she's leaning forward

& smiling a little cleavage & on her blouse
are strawberries, dozens of single

dark red-strawberries, & about this time
when we were falling for one another

she told me she's worked a few summers
in a strawberry-processing factory such

a good job with her friends they
joked & storied the day away while

zillions of strawberries jostled past them
on a belt, & she never lost her taste

for strawberries, so as she picked
off leaves, & stems before the berries

were washed & sugared & packed she'd eat
one after another, the whole shift,

& now we've been married thirty years,
& three years ago she underwent surgery,

a mastectomy, & now of course we fear for her
& all those friends of hers & their children

as strawberries keep arriving to those women
from fields sprayed with DDT

& other poisons they cannot now possibly
Purge from their bodies.

Cindy S. Hochman
Under Anesthesia

[Disclaimer: If you feel this poem is a veritable work of genius, then I will tell you it took hours of precision-like crafting and numerous revisions. If, on the other hand, you think it stinks, then I would remind you that I'm only 7 days post-op, still quite nauseous, in excruciating pain, and largely incoherent.]

> "Jesus was the Son of God
> an unmatchable magician
> he raised Lazarus from the dead
> without a referral from
> his primary care physician"
> Rick Sostchen (my brother)

I.

Doctor, I am lying on your table with my compliant bones
Doctor, soon you will be under my anonymous skin
Doctor, you have reduced me to my lowest common denominator
Doctor, is that a scalpel in your pocket or are you just happy to see me?

II.

Doctor, you are entering my veins with moonshine & Merlot
Doctor, we are more than lovers now, you have known my blood in the Biblical sense
Doctor, row, row, row my boat to some semblance of health
(I will go with the flow)
If my body is a temple, then let us pray.

III.

Doctor, I am curled up in the fetal position, under latex hands and
competent sheets, in a calm room, with a thousand fears, my tongue
tied in a Gordian knot. The cat is throwing up on the floor and I
am furiously licking my paws. The Irish nurse, like a new mother,
whispers "heal" in my cauterized ear. She is laying pink ribbons in
my hair as my palms open like a benign child's. I am dreaming of
lost teeth and follicles dying on the vine. Doctor, I don't see heaven
yet, only some cirrus clouds. This must be cirrus, then. Cirrus of the
liver? Hush, don't cry, God mends all His drunken children.

IV.

What a carnival of organs in here!
Doctor, hurry, London Bridge is falling and Rome is burning!
Doctor, am I drooling all over your slicing hand, are my platelets
in the shape of teardrops? (perfectionist that I am, I am trying to
coagulate for you!)
Doctor, are you discarding the nodules, the pits, the bad seeds, the
dirty parts,
the live wires all along the third rail?
Scoop out the black sin, the badly burned flower
Daughter of suicide and overgrown cells
Doctor, I bequeath to you a hundred secret shames.

V.

Doctor, how much do you charge for a hurt upon hurt upon hurt?
Doctor, is my bloody breast another notch on your surgical belt?
Doctor, how many xx-es have you crocheted with your ugly black
thread?
Tell me how many nodes must a man walk down?
(and is no nodes good nodes?)
Doctor, is that a staple gun in your pocket or are you just happy to
see me?

Philosophical woman, I ache, therefore I am!

VI.

And then the Rich & Handsome Prince and his merry band in scrubs kissed Sleeping Beauty and she woke up and went to work that very afternoon (hungry, but none the worse for wear), with a plastic nipple from K-Mart, some Lenox (Hill) china and a lifetime warranty. You don't have to be Jesus these days to be raised from the dead (as long as you have GHI, Blue Cross/Blue Shield, Medicaid or, in my case, Oxford).

All the world shall be healed!
Bill Clinton shall be healed!
Dick Cheney shall be healed!
Those damned right-wing Republicans (that means you, Sean Hannity) shall be healed!

Melissa Etheridge and Elizabeth Edwards shall be healed!

And yes, boys and girls, even Cinderella, in her size 5 boots, shall be healed
(and will live happily ever after with the surgeon as soon as his divorce becomes final: AMEN!)

Cindy S. Hochman, North Miami, FL. In October 2006 she got married for the first time (at age 49) and relocated from New York to North Miami, Florida. She is a legal assistant and published poet.

"I was diagnosed with breast cancer in 2005 and was treated with surgery, chemotherapy and radiation. It was a big ordeal but I feel I came out of it much stronger."

SaFiya Dalilah Hoskins-Hamm
Can Sir!

Grandpa has Can Sir!

Can Sir! is his will to live.
Can Sir! is his determination to defy the odds.

Can Sir! is Grandpa's magic potion.
Can Sir! is the power of his mind.

Can Sir! daily affirmations motivate Grandpa
and give the family hope about his condition.

Cancer is conquerable.
Can Sir! is Grandpa's mission.

SaFiya Dalilah Hoskins-Hamm, Birmingham, AL, is the Director of Publications & Marketing at Miles College. She earned an M.A. in Communication & Culture ('02) from Howard University. Her professional pursuits include an early career in the entertainment industry with *Radio One, Def Jam Recordings* and BET. In 2006 she published her first novel, *An Infrequent Pairing.* She is a contributor to the *African American National Biography.*

"My poems were inspired by my treasured grandparents Josephine Hamilton-Jones, Calvin Coolidge Jones, Lucy Mae Hoskins-Kincaid and Leroy Kincaid; my beloved father David Earl Hoskins; and a dear friend Olivia 'Fox' Thompson-Larkin; all individuals who showed cancer who's the boss."

Karla Huston
Pencil Test

In 1969, I tucked a pencil
under a breast and when it failed
to cling, I went braless. Brassieres
uncoupled, and everywhere women
waved them like flags, filled
incinerators with nylon and lace.
Later I wore a nursing bra, flap
agape, nipple pulsing while my baby
sucked, and I wrote notes on what not
to forget. One night the neighbor boys
watched through tilted blinds, rubbed
their crotches and spilled their own
milk under a tree in the yard.
Years later when the Wonderbra arrived,
 I tried it, felt cables and wire
cantilevered against my skin
to lift and point even the most
mammogram. As the doctor pulls out
desperate tissue. Today they tell me
they need additional views of a routine,
 the slides, some taken years earlier,
I learn the history of my breasts.
 I stare at the brilliant panels, and there it is,
a transparent web and outlined
in red pencil, the sinister cell, thick
and alarming. As I press fingers
to the circled spot, my worst
fears alight there and flicker.

Karla Huston, Appleton, WI, is the author of five chapbooks of poetry, most recently: *Virgins on the Rocks* (Parallel Press, 2004) and *Catch and Release* (Marsh River Editions, 2005). Her poems, reviews and interviews have been published in *Cimarron Review*, 5 A.M., Margie, *North American Review*, One Trick Pony, Pearl, *Rattle*, and others.

"While I do not have cancer myself, I have had a number of scares. My mother died of colon cancer in August, 2006. My aunt died of multiple myeloma in 2000."

Roy Jacobstein
Parting Conversation

What can you say to your long-
time friend and former lover
who asks do you think much
about death except yes?
She asks because a rare
growth is choking her sacrum.
She tells you she is standing
before a closet door. She means
they are staging her next play
next February and February
is six months away. Her face
shows the sallow full moon
of palliation. You sit other-
wise silent on the back deck.
What you want to say is no.

Roy Jacobstein, Chapel Hill, NC, is a physician working internationally on women's reproductive health. His newest book, *A Form of Optimism* (UPNE, 2006) was selected by Lucia Perillo for the 2006 Samuel French Morse Prize.

Helga Kidder
The Open Drawer

for Betty

The doctors said two years.
She could have crawled into a cave
of self-pity. She could have sailed high
off the Scenic Route driving home late.
She could have taken their savings
on a grand tour around the globe.

If her dreams were too few for an epic,
no one said later she forgot to prepare
for the immediate or the remote.
Dignity was the motif she stitched into
each conversation. She ironed and folded
her days like expensive linens -
her two girls growing toward teenage -
to instill in them years early self-reliance.

She greeted time's limitations graciously.
As if bred Southern. She copied
her destiny's manual — a Xeroxed letter
to family and friends. How to get
everyone a year older.
One more stitch in a hem,
bills paid in the open drawer.
Time to shut outside in.

Helga Kidder, Chattanooga, TN. She received her BA in English from the University of Tennessee and her MFA in Writing from Vermont College. She is co-founder of the Chattanooga Writers Guild and leads their poetry group. Publications include *The Louisville Review*, *The Southern Indiana Review*, *The Spoon River Poetry Review*, *Comstock Review*, *Eleventh Muse*, *Snake Nation Review* and others.

"'The Open Drawer' is about a relative who died of cancer with great dignity."

Emma Lee
A Walk in the Park

She'd never taken the long walk to the park
where summer children used to group and regroup
in cells as friendships waxed and waned;

never sat like this on the bench in the rain
seeing each drop as a frayed thread
as if someone had hacked through it with a blunt knife,

wondering why autumn is the longest season,
remembering the mists on the mammogram results,
thinking what legacy she'd left her own daughters.

Emma Lee, Leicester,United Kingdom. Her poetry collection *Yellow Torchlight and the Blues* has been published by *Original Plus* (UK), *The Journal, Shadow Train, Orbis* and *Borderlines*.

"My poems were inspired by a friend currently undergoing treatment but with a hopeful prognosis and a co-worker who had been in remission but then discovered the cancer had come back, this time fatally."

Emma Lee
Things Not To Say...

You've achieved so much: got your dream house.
I couldn't do that, just up and go to the coast.
When the pain returned, I knew I was going to die.
Might as well make it in my dream house.

Your family have done what they can.
My son's always in tears.
My workaholic daughter merely phones.
My husband had an affair.
My sister's already gone...

I like your handbag.
Here, have it now. I'll empty the contents —
tissues, lipstick, biros, purse —
have it now. He'll forget
and take it to cancer research.

Have you thought what song you'd like at your funeral?
Nothing sentimental. What's left of me
can be scattered out to sea.

How's the weather?
Grey, cloudy and overcast.
It's genetic: my sister, me.
How long's my daughter going to last?

Lyn Lifshin
My Mother Wanted Buttered Bread In Milk

Hours before, she asked for hot
chocolate, wanted me, not any
nurse. The day after fog gulped
branches and we watched films
all afternoon before chicken and
the strawberries I was still smashing
Demerol into. *Butter*, she said,
but thinly, you always do it too
thick, and she drifted back. The
nurse said this was it, whispered,
"Frieda, you're not in pain still,
are you, Honey?" and I, in my own
daze, repeating "I love you,"
cringed when my mother shook her
head, called "Murray, Mama, Lyn,"
the morphine, the last of only two
she'd have put in her, melting. "You
know I do," I said over and over,
the butter melting, a slick on the milk
as time was warped, telescoped.
Cars line the lawn, women with
noodles saying to eat, that I had to do.
Food slid down as sheets did from
my mother's leg, her foot twitching.
"She has no blood pressure," a nurse
said, bread and butter taking my
mother back maybe to the kitchen
table in the house under pines, always
cool near the pantry where there'd be
brownies or yellow cake or lemon
meringue, my mother calling for my
grandmother in that house in her mind,
in the front room were she could see
yellow roses and peonies poke thru,
where the cold pulls away from.

Lyn Lifshin, Vienna, VA. Her most recent books include *Another Woman Who Looks Like Me* (Black Sparrow, 2006) and her prize winning book about the famous, short lived beautiful race horse, Ruffian, *The Licorice Daughter: My Year With Ruffian* (Texas Review Press, 2006). Lifshin's other books include *Before It's Light* (Black Sparrow press,1999-2000), *Cold Comfort, In Mirrors, Upstate: An Unfinished Story* (Foothills Press), *The Daughter I Don't Have*, (Plan B Press), *When a Cat Dies, Another Woman's Story, Barbie Poems, She Was Last Seen Treading Water, Mad Girl Poems, A New Film About A Woman In Love With the Dead*. She is the subject of an award winning documentary film, *Lyn Lifshin: Not Made Of Glass*, available from Women Make Movies. Her web site is www.lynlifshin.com.

"They (poems) are all about my mother and her illness and death in 1990. She lived from May 25, 1911 to August 20 1990....the subject of my mother's bout with cancer has been an obsession."

Lyn Lifshin
Thinking Of That April

My skin still smelling of
rose and jasmine, the bad
news came. Snow and ice
forecaster for a summer
where nothing that mattered
grew anything but smaller.
My mother couldn't swallow.
Soon she couldn't eat.
I thought of the Hau petals
she wouldn't get to see,
the smell of Plumeria
her dress of island colors
couldn't make real. "I can't
even be buried in it," she
frowned. It snowed in Stowe
through May. "Look at the
grackles," my mother said
from a hospital bed, "they
can go anywhere they choose,"
and I thought of the great frigate
birds soaring over the Ke'anae
coast on thermal winds,
hardly flapping, hundreds of feet
upwards, two-foot wing spans,
their feathers weigh the same
amount as their bones,
saw my mother's backbone
hunched bird-like in the only
chair she got to, lighter and
lighter, as if dying
to be lifted into the air

Lyn Lifshin

Dropping the Bottle Of Perfume My Mother Always Wore

on the anniversary of her dying, the
candle for her flickering down
stairs, an eerie light like the
arms of someone drowning. In the
mirror my body seems to be trying

to catch up with her, as if
stripped to the bone it would be
sweeter, close. I'm in a house
that doesn't seem like mine, though
my clothes are in the closet. I want

the smell of her, as Napoleon carried
in a locket the violets that Josephine
always wore, taken from her grave. I
take the Joy out of the drawer where
it's nestled in flannel, and it slips

from my hands, as she did, smashes
on white tile, an explosion of glass.
I try to soak up the gold juice
like someone at a murder trying to sop
up blood. "Shit," I yelp, but only once,

as if I'm in a church or synagogue.
Or because of the day. The bottle
could be me, ragged, in sharp pieces,
empty, holding on to what is gone.
The pale chemise reeks of jasmine

and roses. I take it to my old house,
where once, when we fought and she
said my clothes were slutty, I held
my breath, wondered when
things would change

Lyn Lifshin

Nichols Lodge in the Rain, or, The Night Before My Mother And I Will Take the Ambulance Back to My House, the Last Night I Will Spend Without Her Until the Fall

Corn tassels bending,
hollyhocks, gladiolus
lopped. It's as if the
lettuce had fallen
down for rose zinnias
to kneel on, heads
lowered under the grey.
The Rose of Sharon
dripping, tiger lilies,
beans at the altar of
rain the white spike
flowers hallelujah
up from. Sun flowers
lean against wet wood

On the night before
what I know will be my
mother's last visit, I
try to soak up gladiolus,
violets, all that grows
as my mother just grows
thinner. Jade chrysanthemum
stalks blur Shasta daises,
roses, glistening plums.
Black locusts drip. Rain
flattens sweet peas as
blood grows into the maples
three hours south of
where my mother waits

Green vines, a bracelet
around the wet barnwood
as white bells on the
sills poke up from leaves
that could be shamrocks
or clover. I could use
a 4th leaf spurting in
the grey before what
will be over in a
script I can only
wildly imagine
starts to start

Lyn Lifshin
In My Mother's Last Hours

I write titles for
poems I'll never
write while she's
living in a note
book, shaking as
her eyes roll back
and I feel guilty
I sat on the out
side stoop this noon
while the nurse's aide
changed her. *Mama*
my mother calls out
only a few weeks since
we took the ambulance
down here thru black
eyed susans and she
wanted muffins,
coffee, wanted to
smell the air on
the lake. Her skin
the nurse says is
already mottled. *Lyn*
she gasps, take
me home

Christine Marshall
Johnny Cash Is Dead

When I wake, music reels me
downstairs to my mother

who is laughing, who tells me
I can't write poems but I keep thinking up titles for them

while she works the treadmill
to "I Walk The Line."

He doesn't seem dead in his songs,
she says. It's true: he seems as alive

as she does, dripping sweat
in her spandex,

ponytail bobbing in time.
She doesn't say a word

about my grandfather, who is
visiting, who sits outside

smoking on the porch, his body thin
as a guitar string,

the cancer draining flesh
away, water down the sink.

My mother's spent the past week
pulling family from its graves:

I remember the time Uncle Jay
 cut the toilet seat in two for his half-assed brother.

And when Great-Grandpa slammed his thumb in the car door
and did it again on his way to the hospital.

She can still, sometimes, get
her father to smile — fleeting, emitting

clots of smoke to meet the air
and disappear. She's the only one

who can. Now she thinks
of titles for my poems,

and hums along to songs. When the timer
sounds, my mother stops

the treadmill, climbs
off the track, and turns the music

down. Then she carries
a glass of water outside

to her father — carefully — so
she won't spill a drop.

Christine Marshall, Salt Lake City, UT, is a graduate student in English at the University of Utah. She has been recently published in *Agni*, *Calyx* and *Western Humanities Review*.

"I have lost several close family members to cancer within the last few years."

Christine Marshall
Trying

I. The body

holds life
the way a gutter holds rain, filled
then guttering. Or

the body is life, each cell a whisper
in the chorus singing time. Or

life passes through the body,
slipping past bones
like the wind through reeds. Or

like the drift of cottonwood
seeds in Spring. Or,

or —

II.   At home

after hospice comes,
you no longer eat.

You're tired. Your life
is now a liability.

III   *A tribute*

to you , old man,
can't deliver. How could I
put you on paper?
Janitor, alcoholic, gambler.

No. How about
kind and brave. Or
hands like old trees, faded jeans,
liver spots on your head. No, no.

The body is no less
difficult than the life it pumps, or

is it different at all? Oh
help. A life holds the body?

Like a river holds
silt? Or at least, then, how I hold

on now — how I
can't let go, your life

earth in my fist. And all the time
spent knowing seems

a door, hinged, opening
into silence, leaving

this page —— blackened
with my words.

Karen Nelson
The World Over

The children better pray you don't die in the operating room,
because I'll become an embarrassment and succumb
to traveling the world over, sending elephants home

after riding across African savannas wearing plumes
with men twenty years younger, and then some.
The children better pray you don't die in the operating room,

for I'll make love under the banyan trees, consume
the red hibiscus blooms peering through plums,
traveling the world over, sending elephants home

as heirlooms, drink tea with jam, sweep with a banyan broom,
send giraffes to play with their children, and drums.
They better pray you don't die in the operating room.

I'll follow the animal's home to Kate's room, where they'll eat brome
and roam, while I introduce my latest honey with aplomb.
I'll travel the world over, sending elephants home,

then leave for Australia to watch the ink blue bloom,
looking for coral and shells while drinking rum.
The children better pray you don't die in the operating room.
Traveling the world over, sending elephants home.

Karen Nelson lives in Newton, NH, where she writes poetry, teaches elementary
children, and paints. She taught creative writing through the Newburyport
Adult Education program. Her most recent book "*The Woman You Think I Am*"
was published in 2005. She had poems in *The Larcom Review, Peregrine, Earth's
Daughters, California Quarterly*, and *The Poet's Touchstone*. As a visual artist, she
paints in watercolor and acrylics displaying her work at The *Newburyport Art
Association, Off the Wall gallery, Café de Sienna* and *Starbucks*, in Newburyport,
MA.

"My cancer related poems are about relatives and friends who have had cancer. I have not had cancer. My sister-in-law had breast cancer and my husband had prostate cancer."

Staci L. Nichols
Things That Never Happened

Never been in a plane
crash

Never pulled up to my house to
see the fire fighters putting it out

Never been struck
by lightning

Never heard a doctor say
You'll never walk again

Never got pregnant
in high school

Never was punched during
marriage by my husband

Never spent the night
in jail

But there was
the day Dad interrupted

me wrapping
the Christmas presents

to tell me
he had cancer

Staci L Nichols, Beaumont CA. She minored in Poetry at the University of Redlands, where she studied under renowned poet Ralph Angel. Her work has been published by the *Coal City Review*, *Hot Metal Press*, and the *San Gabriel Valley Quarterly*. Staci currently works at a Field Training Officer/Tribal Officer for a local Indian tribe.

"I think it is great that you are doing this project because one of the editors quoted in *Poet's Market 2007* actually says he doesn't want to read about cancer. He goes on & on about how boring cancer is. When my dad was diagnosed in November, I thought, "Screw that guy! I'm writing about cancer." AND, one of my good friends, a poetry coach & established poet in the Manhattan Beach area, Corine Topal, forwarded me info on your anthology. So word is getting around. Great project. I'm honored just to be considered."

"My Dad is literally THE healthiest guy anybody knows. Never drinks or smokes. He's so young, he has braces! Eats only weird stuff from the health food store, works out religiously, for recreation kicks guys' butts half his age in Tae Kwon Do tournaments, etc...But he owned a truck tire business for 30 years. Every day he sat in a warehouse the size of a football field, filled 3 stories tall with truck tires. Each tire has about 20 gallons of petroleum product in it. They believe his cancer (pancreatic) may be caused by exposure to petroleum products."

Staci L. Nichols
Two Months

What he didn't know
holding her blue-eyed baby
fat that
grabbed for this ears and hair

is that one day
he would get on
a plane
and tell that baby
twenty-seven years old

nothing is wrong
not want to ruin
her big second
date wait
until the right
moment

a moment that
to this day
is still hanging in
the air over
the living room couch

when he would
have to tell her
if the chemo
doesn't work the
doctors say

two months

Pat Parnell
Whispers From the Darkness

(The speaker is a kidney cancer, before it was discovered.)
(kidney cancer surgery, 9/12/05)

In this womb that is not a womb,
I grow as the slow years pass.
Unrecognized, I share your strength.
Absorb your knowledge, quietly, steadily.
Cause no problems.

My bulk bulges from your kidney
like the foot of a fetus
poking against the abdominal wall. Your dreams
are of pregnancy, of nursing a child: your body telling you
I am here, milking you, but you do not understand.

Sometimes, with my spoke-wheel configuration,
I see myself as an octopus:
the lump of my head the wheel's hub,
my beak in your flesh, gulping,
my tentacles reaching out in a circle to hold and hug.

Or sometimes I see myself as a 17 year locust,
sucking your sustenance in the darkness,
my great lumpy cicada shape buried deep.

When I am ready, I will burst open my shell like the cicada.
My little ones I will send out of myself
to find their own flourishing.
My babies will burrow into your vulnerability.
There they will grow as I have grown,
and so the cycle continues.

I am what I was conceived to be,
perfect in form and function.

Pat Parnell, Stratham, NH. I am currently working on a third collection of poetry, *Of Masks and Mirrors*. My poems have appeared in area and national journals and anthologies, and I serve as a featured reader and workshop presenter of poetry.

"My sister Ruth had surgery about 10 years ago for endometrial cancer. Her oldest daughter, Sarah, had surgery for cancer in the uterine wall. Both Ruth and Sarah have periodic checkups to make sure the cancer has not reappeared."

"The poem 'Whispers from the Darkness' was written before my surgery, when I was trying to understand what was going on inside my body. It is written in the first person, with the cancer as the speaker, and the time is before the cancer was discovered."

Tzynya Pinchback
Healer Woman

wellness done come to town dressed as an old woman
wide-hipped and black/sauntering up the road to my door/carrying
unfiltered honey/cloves/and a plant for my windowsill

a season ago i kept watch for her/when God was teaching my body
to clean house/pin to the line some sadness/sickness/any ole thing
planned to sit for a spell and weigh down a spirit

and here i see myself/of earth/breath/fire and water/
of sea glass and stone/cracked rock and fine jewel/
creeping over mountain/standing tip-toe/sweeping the fine line of the
moon/
palming the full-bellied sun

with these hands/this voice/i stand/sing

Tzynya Pinchback, Roswell, GA, grant proposal writer by day, poem-maker
by night. Author of *EveSongs* (*Paladin*, 1996); *HoneyChild* (2007) a free
ebook; and *Gypsy: Courtesan in Prose and Poem* (work in progress). She
served as *MindSkin* columnist for *Chaotic Dreams Online* (2005-2007); *Cafe
Afrikana* columnist for *Momentum Ezine* (2005); and contributing writer/
music & events reviewer for *Smooth Jazz Magazine* (2004-2006).

"My poem was written for two very dear friends, one who is a new survivor
and one who left us in winter."

Kim Ben-Porat
The Esophagus

There it was, on the pathologist's
cutting board like a cucumber.
Red, as pepper, fatter
than expected: pimpled with tumors.

I didn't want to look at her disease,
her anorexia, her bulimia, her bad humors.
So I walked around, denial stirring
my own ulcer until it boiled.

I peeked through my brother's professional
readiness, past my sister's breasts
and around my father's attempt
to steady his own gut, then vomit.

Forced to witness the insult of disease
on an innocent organ created for the sole purpose
of transporting food, I leaned against the wall
and considered the sea.

I called up the water and salt and the pebbles
of Venice. I remembered the juggler on the corner
and the man under the paper mumbling
when I walked the dog last week.

I ran into my lungs and breathed,
breathed in the spirit of sand,
heard the voices beneath me until I was calm
to view again the piece of my mother on a plate.

Kim Ben-Porat, Raanana, Israel, holds a MFA from Bennington College, has two novels, Israeli based, in English, looking for publishers, grew up in Boston and moved to Israel in 1976, at the age of 17, currently lives outside Tel-Aviv with her four teenagers.

"My mother survived 60 days in the ICU in Los Angeles after 10 hours of surgery when her esophagus was removed and replaced. Two years later she drives and swims again. My father, three siblings and I never left her side during this ordeal and she was prayed for by friends and relatives on a daily basis. She survived clinical death which is considered a miracle by the staff in the ICU."

Liz Rosenberg
Another Thing She Gave

In Memory of Becky Levy

In the hospital I looked for the face
that was my friend's, and found it floating
like a full moon; bloated, calm
smiling over her bald sheets
and the thin white blanket,
the swivel table and the tray;
her left arm partly amputated, wrapped in gauze
held up like a flag of truce—

I looked into the face
that was my friend's
while doctors and nurses raced along the halls.
All hard at work,
the medicine still at war with that
disease which always loses in the end....
though sometimes only in the very end.
We talked about our young boys, going around

together as vampires for Halloween,
both of us smiling ruefully.
Then dinnertime's trays began to crash outside the door,
-and she and I in the square white room,

removed from all that—

for a few minutes alone,
in the face of it,
were strangely together at peace.

Liz Rosenberg, Binghamton, NY. Her first husband, the late novelist, John
Gardner, was considered completely cured of colon cancer at the time of his death

in a motorcycle accident. She herself is a survivor of cervical and skin cancer. She teaches English at the State University of NY at Binghamton and has published three books of poems, two novels and dozens of books for young readers, including five award-winning poetry anthologies.

Liz Rosenberg
The Blue-Flowered Bell

No more New Years for you, beloved,
whose grave has no monument.
The Crab is scuttling across the sky.
I am thinking of the clumsy blue ornament
we clipped with hospital shears
and the old Jewish woman,
a jaunty basket over her arm
who visited her husband at his machines,
of the white-soled nurses with tubes and instruments
who made you cry out
till I paced the halls on fire
because in that place there was still
something holy: TO PRESERVE HUMAN LIFE,
preserve human life— the voice that is elsewhere
unspoken or lost. We spent that winter
near wharfs and waterfronts,
past the information desk, corridor,
stench of cafeteria, and on up the elevator
studying one Matisse print till our eyes
fell out, till the colors shrank up,
and still I remember the death-smell
that clung to your bandages,
uncoiling the gauze
from the hole in your belly,
adjusting the I.V.—
as long as I sat near you, I still believed
you could not die.
Driving home in the dark
past Sears, a cop would flash his lights at me,
a signal mine were off again—
blind, dark mole of a car creeping home.

That year you survived
we hung the crooked bell on the tree.

At four a.m. the halls were quiet,
the nurses' station quiet too, the snow rang
on the old green dome like thunder, and the saint in the lobby
stood guard, enormous, while human guards dreamt.
You slept under damp sheets.

I sat next to you, giddy to welcome the new year,
holding my gifts from you: three bars
of scented soap, two prs. socks, a knitted thing
for under motorcycle helmets, kaleidoscope,
bandages, peppermints, and aspirin.

Liz Rosenberg
Valentine's Day At Johns Hopkins Hospital

The elevator sinks
to the first floor
where the guard taps his pencil on a wooden desk.
The halls are vacant
though this afternoon we saw mother and child,
both in blue robes, holding hands,
and earlier still the worried crowd
pushing for the doors. Drunks and
nurses, the black man big as a rock
whose bulk was cut off at the hip--
all have gone. In the cafeteria a woman eats
a late meal, rummaging through a paper bag.
There's snow in the yard.

In the yard, the city bus steams.
Late couples take the dark seats
at the back. Snow slides
under the heavy wheels.
Above, the sky's a scratched, smudged yellow.
At each rise
of the wheels, and fall, I'm drawn from you.

Last night the hammock moon slung
light on the rug.
You gathered me up,
your hair like water on my cheek.
Now I walk through snow
that melts on my lips as it falls.
When I left, you lay
on white sheets,
beautiful, your hands square and hard.
Dogs circle loose in the street,
follow me halfway home, then turn.
I want to go back,

force some burning wish on the stars,
seize you with this mouth, but I do
as you would have me do.
Face my back to the darkness and walk home.

Liz Rosenberg
Waiting For a Sick Friend

Let the maple rave
and the light fall
on the last bent grass,
Let the willow spin its gold to straw.
Let the yellow moth rest.

May the sky in its blue enamel,
burn under the slow-moving cloud.
Let a good day surround him.
Let the pigeons sing their dull bright songs
as they peck at the glass
like exotic dancers, offering their green necks.

For I waited an hour at a sidewalk café
For my friend to come, my panicked heart drumming,
And fire chasing the blood from my finger ends
as I feared each passing, sick, drawn,
dessicated face was his;
and when one man, a walking skeleton,
with a patch of black hair, drew near
I nearly passed out

as jauntily down the street
lit on one half of his body by sun,
the other striped in shadow, like a motley
fool, my friend came, my ordinary, handsome
dying Nathan, and sat down by me
to drink the shining half-moon of his tea.

Liz Rosenberg
Couple On Hospital Elevator

With grime-blackened fingernails
he touches her face with the back of his hand
while she makes that long, slow, secretive swipe
that wipes away weeping.

Flat on her back on the hospital gurney, her hair stubbled short,
the IV bag swaying beside her like a giant tear.
They fix their eyes together on the floor number display

watching it fall; then, still bending toward her,
he follows her into the lobby,
saying goodbye. And how shall we stand it,
how shall we bear it,
what good can come of this?

I beg you to send them health, Lord!
—or if not health, comfort;

and if not even comfort, then brandish a radiance
from your broken sparks
brilliant enough
to make these sorrows possible to bear.

Helen Ruggieri
Leading Causes Of Death

Heart Disease

Most die of broken hearts,
smashed vessels, constricted avenues
they let go wide-eyed
regretting their last meal
when they realize the rhythm
is gone and the silence
fills them up.

Cancer

Their secret nature
turns against them,
life gets pregnant
with death.
They cut and cobalt
until your bald pate glows
and your raggedy skeleton
can't sit upright;
they kill you to save you and
take it slow until there's a hole
in your life as big
as a grave and they say
try it on,
see what you think.

Stroke

If you wake up, you're wordless;
you have the picture but not the name.
There's no way of saying.
That which you were, that deep
vocabulary more faithful than a lover,
has abandoned you.

Accidents

Falling,
 from high places,
 asleep at the wheel,
 off the ladder,
the long, slow,
arc we describe
as we enact our last fall.

Pneumonia/Lung Disease

The lungs give up, fill up,
say the hell with it.
It's too much work to go on;
we drown in our own exhaustion .

Deabetes

Comes thirsty —
dying blind
dying by parts
dying sweetly.

Alzheimer's

forget it
forget the world
forget the self
forget the word
forget.

Suicide

They give up on themselves,
won't wait;
select their own moment.
These are the ones
strangled by grief,
who choke on exhaust,
slice open the thin
vein of time.

Helen Ruggieri, Olean, NY. Helen Ruggieri has a book of short prose pieces, *The Character for Woman*, from *foothillspublishing.com* and a book of poetry, *Glimmer Girls*, from *mayapple.com*.

"My father and my husband both died of cancer. Hell of a way to go."

Elizabeth Schott
Minnesota

This urge to take my child
back to the place he
has never seen, it must be
biological. There is, after all,
nothing there for him but graves.

My mother's grave on what
was once a gently rolling hill
in the countryside on the way
to the beach, (we used to beg her
to take us) now surrounded
by subdivisions. I could not find it
for all the snow, lay down and,
swinging my arms and legs,
made an angel.

The two graves of my father's
parents. There lies rotting
everything they never gave us,
inlaid in hardwood and polished like brass.
The Canada geese waddle through,
squawking.

The graves of the beloved grandparents
are there too, and here, in the ashes
of the water, the soil, the air.
We do not need to travel to find them.

And the living grave,
the one that does not decay
or give way because fresh
blood pumps through it daily:
my father's heart.

Elizabeth Schott, Santa Barbara, CA, has a doctorate in Art History from UC Berkeley and taught art history and writing for 12 years at Berkeley, USC, and UCSB. She was awarded a Fulbright Scholarship to the Netherlands, as well as a Mellon Fellowship for study at the University of Leiden. She has also won a SBWC fellowship through the Community of Voices Poetry Contest. Her work has appeared or is forthcoming in numerous literary journals including *Mindfulness Bell, South Carolina Review, The Handmaiden, Illuminations* and several anthologies. She currently works as a Poet in the Schools and writes for the Santa Barbara Independent.

"My mother died of breast cancer in 1984 when I was 17 years old."

Carol Schwalberg
On Dodging Bullets

Pork-pied and angry, you came with Wanda.
"The hysterectomy went well,"
I told them. "My husband said I dodged a bullet."

Wanda smiled in encouragement, but you looked glum.
"You can't keep on dodging bullets," you said.
"Some day one will catch up with you."
Wanda's eyes looked desperate.

You died of Kaposi's sarcoma.
Did Wanda know then?
Will I know soon?

Carol Schwalberg, Santa Monica, CA. Her poems have appeared in *Black Buzzard Review, West, Black River Review, Yet Another Small Magazine, The Sunday Suitor, Krax* (U. K.) and *New Voices Anthology*. Her short stories have appeared in *Wordplay, Fair Lady* (South Africa), *Ita* (Australia), and several anthologies.

"I was diagnosed with endometrial cancer 17 years ago. The endometrium is the mucous membrane of the womb. Surviving cancer gave life more zest and it is that zest which informs my poetry."

Hannah Shr
Bodies Can Move This Way

All I can think about is the hospital waiting room
How it didn't reek at all
And how the black receptionist called me "guuurrrrllllll".

We ordered Chinese food at half past nine
And we gorged ourselves to replace our grief
But in the end I still felt like shit
And I knew the black doctor was watching me;
I couldn't even hold in my stomach I was so full.

We were there from 4 to 10.
The family gathered around me and braided my hair.
They argued and laughed over Andy
And his confusion at the art of braiding.

I was the only one to see her pass us,
My mother.
Her body in the gurney, lying so small
A plastic oxygen mask on her face.
And I slipped away.

We passed the time watching fat celebrities
compete to lose weight
I claimed to be calm and unalarmed,
Even when my grandmother started to cry
I treated her like a nervous child.

But when for the first time in half a year my father called me
He apologized. And wished my mother luck.
I didn't tell him how much that meant to me.
I didn't want my family to hear.
But later at 11:00
In front of the computer,
For the first time since my mom told me she had cancer
I cried.

Hannah Shr, San Francisco, CA. Hannah Shr will be published in a love anthology by Candlewick Press.

"My mother is a cancer survivor."

Kelly Sievers
One Life

The last snow
came early that morning.
In a hushed moment
he stood in robe and slippers
with the morning paper
tucked under his arm.
He saw how snow forgave
the sagging porch, exposed
a balance in the dogwood,
humored the wild tamarisk
he had trimmed for forty years.
The snow held no shadows---
bridal wreath, camellia,
even the raffish fig,
were innocent with light.

Kelly Sievers, Portland , OR, is a Nurse Anesthetist with Kaiser Permente. Her poems appeared in *Prairie Schooner*, *Seattle Review*, *Poet Lore*, *The Bridge*; *The Greensboro Review*, and other.

"'One Life' was written as a tribute to a neighbor. I knew he had been diagnosed with liver cancer. One morning I was sitting at my table looking out the window at the new snowscape. I saw my neighbor paused on his front porch. He died within a few months of his diagnosis."

Micki W. Simms
Rumi's Pole Dance

On the second Sunday of Lent
the Christmas cactus burst
into late bloom with one
giant bud exploding
and a second coming on.
That day my mother began her
active dying process.
By Wednesday night, the bud
assumed the shape of an angel in flight,
circling the ceramic pot— round
and round it went
as though leading something.
Thursday morning while
crossing the threshold
from this world to the next,
the smaller bud began opening seraphic-wise
with the giant guiding angel now in pursuit.
Twice daily as I face west and read
Mourner's Kaddish, I wonder,
could it be symbolic of
my father coming to lead his bride home
as he led her to the altar so many years ago?

Micki W. Simms, Houston, TX. She has had numerous poems and several essays
published including *Brigit's Journal*, and *Reflections*.

"The poems included in these submissions are related to the months before
and soon after my mother's death from metastatic breast cancer March 9, 2005.
Although they do not deal with issues relating specifically to the disease process,
they speak to the grief process as I experienced it prior and subsequent to my
mother dying, to the death of her best friend (whom I had know all my life) who
died eight months later to the day. I walk in fear praying that her fate will not
become mine."

Linda Simone
Stations Of the Cross

Station One (condemned)

Your Pilate, a doctor, white-clad,
says the disease sleeping these many years
has resurfaced, that, *no,*
you aren't crazy, the pain
the ragged raw spot that zips
through your bladder, is real.

You stand before him, still whole,
hands behind your back,
gunmetal hair, clear hazel eyes,
still able

to piss like a kid,
like the cop you once were
beat back 3 times by crimes
of nature — cancer

back, not arrested.
Can you walk on water, too?
This time, will you make
it to the hilltop? How do you silence
your cry?

Station Two (bearing)

When the terrible weight is laid on you
again
you rise, ace surgery,
chemo drip twice a week —
almost a pillar of strength.
Childlike, you don't believe the story ends.
I feel great, you say. I answer

the two of you — the dark-haired man,
full-bodied, full of life
and the one, faded gray — with a kiss.
The mass has found your lungs,
Coughs, your punctuation.
Megadoses of promise in a new drug.
In a zip, they say you'll lose your hair
go bald like your two brothers
who got the bad genes —
or the good ones.

Station Three (first fall)

You've hardly begun and already
We are coming apart, dividing like the cells inside you.
We clink glasses,
your wife barely mouthing the toast.

In the unforgiving white lights
of Christmas, her eyes,
yours — shadowed by pain.
Not just for 2004, you say, *but for many years.*
We say *yes, yes,* but don't believe

you believe. Tonight, renouncing the ritual wine,
you are someone we don't know
dark

and farther from us.
I imagine thoughts
that zip through your head
relive decades.

Station Four (mother)

On your raw canvas, the line
has moved closer.
I visualize the invisible
careening like meteors,
zipping into small galaxies
in your lungs.

Will your dead mother absorb
explosions of pain
And like mothers do, will she live in you,
a thin white voice that won't dissolve?

Station Five (carrying)

Loneliness a big black presence,
two gravities that zip us toward opposite poles.
We ache to do some
thing. But what? Listen? Talk?

Even trekking with a woman for 47 years
doesn't mean much on this last leg.
This path, big enough for one,
shifts from all the footsteps
before — the journey
we are born to.
I've never died before, you say.
Will sense break through? And, in the end,
will we finish knowing, then?

Station Six (wiping)

Your face a mask
left on batik cloth — eyes sunken,
smile zipped a tight grimace

pain-splotched skin,
hair, sparse white strands.

We watch The Belmont on TV.
Your wife tells you
she dreamt of your dead mother-in-law,
waving lottery tickets, smiling.

That's a good sign, she says.
I want to believe that too. Me
to whom my mother never comes in dreams
bearing lottery tickets or anything at all.
Me who doesn't believe in luck.
I want to cover you in four-leaf clover,
a hutch of rabbit feet.

Station Seven (second fall)

The benchmark month: visit to the Seer-scan,
hope rising like cream.
You've endured the siege
zip-locked in bedrock fatigue.
On Easter, the faithful praise another Rising.

We await results, whisper *He looks pretty good…
better than last week.*

One by one, we seek you out
give the longer hug
ask *Do you need anything?*
Two days later from market aisle,
I can no longer wait to call.

Not so good. Your wife's voice like lead.
The tumor's grown.
On to plan B. I have no words,

yearn to thrust raw meat like missiles
shatter bottles of wine vinegar
watch them spatter on C-Town linoleum
like blood.
Instead I say *I love you,*
buy turkey for supper,
ground and pale.

Station Eight (the women)

Here are the ones who do the small things
wipe away pus, tears, blood,
always busy
scrubbing, rubbing,
cooking, joking,
calling family and friends,
waking, zipping up emotions in a cocoon,
in silence, wailing.

They are so good at what they do
you hardly notice anymore—
daughter, wife,
pillars of your life

raising you up
else you come
crashing down.

Station Nine (third fall)

They say you'll get stronger in the rehab place,
push therapies to make you walk again.
We sit on the patio like it's your own backyard.
Clown Fish zip across the pond,
bring no smiles. You still joke as you shift
trying to find a spot where the tumor isn't.

More visitors — are we helping?
Is solitude your choice?

Home for Father's Day, you look strange
in your daughter's house, smaller,
need to retreat — like you're practicing good-byes.
You struggle down the front stairs,
bolstered by two brawny sons
The next day,

a set-back. BP plummets. A sudden weakness.
Back to Sloan. Reevaluated — like a mortgage.
Another long weekend before the scans come back.
Time to move to the final stop
before the final stop.
We cry. You're relieved.

Station Ten (stripped)

Under a robe of pink *fleurs de lis*
a large blue diaper is zipped closed.
Your back, now a mountain range of bone.

You wait for Joe, my husband with the bad back
to play Mick to your Rocky, coax you from bed,
cheer on your lap around the hospital floor.

From outside your door, I watch you
end this round, push the silver walker
legs sliding slow, steady
and I almost hear
the crescendo of trumpets.

Station Eleven (nailed)

You still go to work, still to chemo:
the poison, the bathroom, functions
that burn and there's no controlling it.

For your wife extra worry, extra laundry.
And for you the constant unzipping,
zipping, unzipping — no other option.
Life, such as it is.

Station Twelve (dying)

Now you can get anything
You want: steak, lobster,
Drugs. You want nothing
But to walk the high school track alone
Cheer on your grandson's ballgame from the stands.
You are center stage
The object of pricks and wipes, of monitors
And shifts in position.
We've already forgotten the pitch
Of your voice, stare at the pitch
Of your chest. Wait.

Station Thirteen (taken down)

You enjoy this day,
a good day.
In the restaurant, we break bread
forks zipping across plates to sample each others' fare.
We plan for a birthday celebration
one month away

We all make sacrifices
to be here.

Back at your house, karaoke.
You palm the mike
belt out a song with gusto,
grin like a rock star,
even manage fancy footwork—
you're a gift to us. We laugh
at your old self,
greedy for the relief.

Station Fourteen (entombed)

Zip-a-dee-doo-dah. The three of you, brothers,
partners in crime,
as you grew up.

Now you alone
hang between the two,
wondering who nailed
the wiseass title
above your head.

You accept the one who grieves
from far away in his own way.
The younger wears his pain
dead-center,
wishes he could take all that bad,
zip it up out of sight,
give in return a fresh set of new hopes
to wear
before the last breath of spring
turns gray.
Zip-a-dee-ay.

BE II: JC Rising

Always at the head of our table,
now, in 100 photos spread across it,
you look out at us —
a constellation of smiles —
from your Florida honeymoon,
under your patrolman's hat,
from a blue Aruba beach.

Like the new moon, you rise
in your wife's eyes
the way your children move
in your grandchildren's crescent lips, cleft chins.

You ascend in words
that flood our mouths:
  "Remember the eaters club…"
    "Remember that cruise…"
      "Remember when Jerry…"

Still, you light the night —
a single star that arcs our sky.
Your trail gives us reason
to look, look up
to smile.

Linda Simone, New York, NY. Linda Simone's chapbook, *Cow Tippers*, won the
2006 Shadow Poetry Chapbook Competition. Her poems have appeared in *Review
Americana, Cezanne's Carrot, Westview, Potomac Review, Essential Love: Poems
about mothers and fathers, daughters and sons*, en(compass) and other journals and
anthologies. She serves as faculty advisor for *Inkwell*, at Manhattanville College.
Look at www.lindasimone.com.

"The chapbook structure is inspired by Barnett Newman's series of paintings called *The Stations of the Cross: Lema Sabachthani*. This series consists of 14 Abstract Expressionist paintings plus a final painting titled "Be II." The paintings, the only true series for Newman, represent variations on a single cry. They are really about human endurance in the face of terrible suffering. These paintings, housed in the National Museum in Washington, D.C., moved me in a powerful and visceral way. I was inspired by Newman's signature *zip*, a line that, depending on how you view the painting either pulls two sides together or pushes them apart. I worked to emulate this by challenging myself to incorporate some form of the word *zip* into each poem. My intention is to capture the experience of being a bystander — emotional, hopeful, and helpless — along each of the *station's* of my two brothers-in-law's journeys battling cancer. In the end, my hope is that, in art, we can find some comfort, understanding and acceptance."

Carole Sineni
That Last Morning

I loved holding your hand
It was warm and swollen soft.
You were all mine again,
my baby.

I think it was a clear day through
the curtain;
sunny, like any spring day.
The corners of your eyes were wet.
I don't know if that was a tear
or just the way the body begins to die.
I think it was tears, Karen.

Who knows what for,
there were so many reasons—
maybe because the children had become
so quiet, maybe because love, love that
erases everything
except you in the vast
white bed
is the greatest pain of all.

Maybe it was just tears for your hair;
all those curls just blowing away
caught in the trees, stolen
by the winds of March.

Suddenly you struggled, searching
for air,
your mutilated breast heaving,
old voodoo death shaking his rattle.

For one impossible moment
you opened your eyes and raised your head

and looked straight at me
so amazed.
What did you see, my little Karen?
Did you see God? Did you see God?

Carole Sineni
At the Moment Of Death My Mother Comes To Karen

Lifting its shadow,
now the curtain (which is lily
white
sky and trees translucent)

billows and sucks in

like the breath of someone
who will disappear
before your eyes.

Breath
clotted with lily white cotton

of someone who
is sky and trees translucent.

At just that moment of the curtain
lifting, cumulus nimbus,
she, through the membrane translucent,

saw 1942:
the backyard, the clothesline
held up by poles, the pure white
of the summer
curtains puffing and slapping
in the upstate wind,

my mother, coiled auburn haired,
bending and pinning,
bending and pinning.

Carole Sineni, Charleston, SC, was born in Buffalo, NY. She received her B.A. from Connecticut College and her M.A. from SUNY at Buffalo. Carole was a columnist for the now defunct *Courier Express* newspaper in Buffalo; an editor of the literary magazine *Escarpment*; and was nominated twice for the Pushcart Prize. She is presently working on a volume of poetry to benefit victims of breast cancer and their families, and has a chapbook, *Liebestod* forthcoming from Pudding Press. Her work has appeared in *Nimrod, The Bitter Oleander, Pleiades, Catfish Stew, The Pittsburgh Quarterly* and others. Carole is co-editor of *Hotmetalpress*. Carole Sineni (Carolina) is a poet who lost her daughter Karen Fredericks in 2004 to breast cancer and finds Karen's voice in poetry.

Carole Sineni
New Music For My Daughter

(*for two voices*)
of breast cancer 5/22/04
And In Memorium Adam Ross
  Hari Kari 1988

In heaven

       At the concert of "New Music"
     it rushes like tsunami from
   the violin, cello, the flute, the flute.
   We are all drowning.

Karen is swimming naked
with Adam.
    The cello,

Laughing, among the rocks,
     out of the chaotic swaying and swelling
     lyrical, romance and

they navigate by a swinging electric
light
to his father's kitchen,
where he committed
Hari Kari.

     its passion like flame flower

She does not ask him,
 "Why?"   *possesses us.*

but touches the small
bleeding place
and tastes.
    Red is the color of my true love's blood

He and I are made of mud.
"Adam."

Her children,
with their stained
eyes,   Like a cobra the saxophone sways,
                          one ruby eye
                          undulating as it muses upon
                          the unimaginable sorrow
                          of innocence.

sit at the dinner table
eating lemon pie.
"It is good."   The marimba, the cymbals and sticks,
                          signify nothing.
                          Dust in my mouth.
                                         He spat into the dust and made Adam.
                          DUST.

the little boys tell Phoebe.
                          Where is the God of my mother?
                          Her beauty was the sweetness
                          in our mouths.
                          Dust.

And Karen and Adam
taste.

In that place in the forest
                                         The piano is a beast who lies
down
                              with the children
                              in the dark fragrant grass
                              to watch the stars.
where we used to go,
the darkness, mysterious
with light,
surrounds like Karen's

wild hair.
                              How mystical is the moon.
                    Is it not forbidden to sing its name;
                    LOVE, seven veiled in beauty.
  There wild irises grow.

Adam bends on a slender stem
and plucks one flower for Karen.
She holds it out to me.
                    The waves lift us; we hear the screaming
                    sea birds, the Iraqi woman who tears her hair,
                    bodies of exotic children piled among
                    the minor lament, covered with flies…
                    three quarter notes.
They touch my tears
and taste.

In childhood sleep
the children hear
the delicate song,
the lullaby, she dreamed.
From far away she sings
that beauty is more

                              Over and over again I asked
                    you to play the little piano piece
                    of Bach until you knew that I
                    had guessed your secret face
                    and then you ran away among
                    the apple branches to press
                    your tears against Adam.

than pain.

Far, far away,
Karen's sweetness lives.
And the children,
soft,

soft as a breath,   *Saxophone, cello, violin, making*
a terrifying

sickle. Tsunami!
Passionate curve rising and falling,

and the music
stops, and stops,
the flute....
She was the sweetness
in our mouths.

are touched
and taste.

Carole Sineni
Finding Persephone

               I stand at the edge
so stilled as the star still dark.

Your voice shivering across the creek,
 across marsh, across bay

strumming the steel chords of the glass bridge.

 Looking for you, I hear your voice.
                  The medium said you sing to me.

Searching for you; wandering, lurching,
but coming back south

and dark and the scent of jasmine bush
at the porch.

               I was not afraid to be lost

as if it were not serious,
as if together we could laugh at the black thread you unwind;

              "Persephone!"

               flinging into moss wind your name, as the scent of
ocean,
damp earth and jasmine opening.

Looking for you, your voice singing, jeweled as pomegranate, deep
as lovers and the scent of jasmine

floats away like childish laughter,
sifts through the cold earth of my hands.

Carole Sineni
Lullaby for Karen

1. Music falters as in Schubert, in the romantic
hesitance. As if the heart...
this gasp of women loving
roses as if they could exist.

2. Sea voices sighing of women
as curved
sloping beaches
low tied to the horizon,

3. Things to be found
in the Perfect Presence Of All Things which is to say
the Overhushing of God's Dreaming

4. Wanting, as if a howl inside the waltz
of butterflies.

5. No, the dead do not eat or dream.

6. They slip off the silk rustling and look
on.

7. They do not understand tears or sorrow
in their high petal place.
Their beauty falls to their shoulders.

Carole Sineni
Tie Her Silk Ribbon

In Memory of My Daughter Karen

It is rose,
that filament, fine canyon of belief and apprehension,

that butterfly out of sight over the sea glass waves,
grey, and the butterfly dark, iridescent wing
as in a locket, or strange antique broach.

That distance within nothing, as when hands
touch and their speech is palpable.

Magic as in faith.

The jubilant cosmos
is
no more
or less.

In these you are alive;
and listening as the quiet listens
to itself.

Hear, as though the sea seems to fall and rise,
seems to separate sound at its fragile middle

vibration.

  *

Sometimes the stunning violence of disbelief
the incandescent opening of that brutal star
illuminating the space, the fragment

of where I am just then, just reaching for a book,
just looking in the mirror to pin back my hair,

just the melody intimating yearning over my shoulder
looking back, not daring to look.

Promise me you will not go no matter what.
Your soft hand.

Carole Sineni
We Were Good At It

The first time I came after the news
and I asked "What can I do, honey?"
you said "Just lie down with me, Mom."
We fell asleep, my arm across you.

Most of the time I wanted to just
scoop you up in a receiving blanket
and take you away with me to some
soft place.
You said, "People die you know, Mom."
I said, "Yes, but not now, honey."

I wanted to talk to you about God
and about all the things that no one
can imagine because this was a movie.
You looked away and opened your
beautiful lips to be fed.

But before things got that bad,
you could remember each turn
on the way to your appointments
while I drove those pretty Bucks County
roads.
You were dizzy and your face
was set as you walked holding on
to me down the corridor to the elevator.

That wig was a dead giveaway.

Allison Smythe
The Way a Day Can Break
for Cathy McMillan

After weeks of cold indifference the sun
came out, like a lost friend, the air
tinged with memories of other thawings.
We were younger then. Rare snow limned
the campus and we, unschooled in such
reversals of forecast, abandoned
books for bathing suits just two days later.
We sunned in sudden heat, weightless
as the songs blasting from our portable radios.
We were radiant, buoyed by all we did
not yet know, the skin of the world still intact
like a ripe, unbitten peach. The future tied
with a bow— our best, unopened
present. We gleamed in scentless
sweat, our bodies dazzling in the sun's
brilliance, so bright on our lids
that when we opened our eyes we could see
nothing before us.

Cathy, does your daughter remember you, only
two that first and last time I saw her? The cells
in your womb multiplied in perverse
accounting: your child thrived inside
your dying. Somewhere now she invents
your likeness. I would like to tell her
how we rode around Lubbock with the top
rolled down and *Journey* turned up, how you
pointed at white tipped cotton fields shouting, *Look,
they're growing wool!*; about our double
date to the Hairy Buffalo party where we
discovered you can't taste Everclear in punch.
How we shared hairstyles and heartbreaks, played

cards and baked cookies, saran wrapped toilet bowls
in the dorm. How you laughed. That summer
we caravanned home in matching, secondhand
Toyotas, glassy days of skiing on the shimmering
lake before evening's slow surrender. I would like
to hand her those days—to give her you—
before
you carried all you would leave behind.

Allison Smythe, Rocheport, MO.

"This poem is in honor of a close friend from college. She died at 36 of ovarian
cancer not long after delivering her first child. She was diagnosed while
pregnant."

Penny Sutton
Bye Folks — Love From Trisha

It's sort of, well … kind of … fatal.
Just thought it was my ailing heart;
breathlessness, like the flowing tide,
cuts short my daily shoreline walk.
It's back; "liver metasteses," they said.

My tumbled thoughts, a foaming sea.
Spring-clean, tidy — while I still can.
Each day a blessing; sea, salt air,
shining sands lift my anguished soul.
Life's drawing in, "maybe three weeks," they said.

Oh Wonder Drug, chemo, hopes raised.
What? Another birthday? More time?
Tears flow and dry, failing body,
frenzied mind, flagging spirits. And
yet, "You could have a few months more," they said.

Friends gather for my living wake;
Speeches — loyal wife, special mum,
favourite sister, rolled into one;
email, snail mail, telephone calls
"We're here to share your precious life," they cried.

My moods, like anchored harbor boats
bob up and down; then, a stillness
glistening in the moon-glade.
Anxiety, chaos, becalmed.
Tall ships waiting to sail away; I sighed.

My resting place, beside the sea,
Lemonwood rustles in the breeze,
a bench where folk might rest and smile,
and stare beyond the ebbing tide.

No more time; at just sixty-one I died
surrounded by your love; I watched, you cried
as I drifted away on the final tide.

Penny Sutton, Garnswllt, Ammanford, South Wales, UK. She spent the first 38 years of her life in Africa. Her two sons were born in Zambia and spent their early years there prior to her husband's untimely death. Published works include: *Clumber*, *ISA's*, *Star Letter*.

"Should this be published, it would be my way of thanking Trisha for everything she gave to me during our friendship and, sadly, at the end of her life, too. She is remembered with great fondness by all who knew and loved her."

Jackie Swift
Diminished in C

And I do feel less — somehow
Smaller, diminished.
Defeated by this world.
As if the new job and the disease have taken too much from me.

They have stopped me
Kept me in check
Corralled
Constrained
Contained

Such that I have taken steps backwards.
Inwards
Where the courage, the largeness and the loudness that is me
is loosened from me
Taken from me.
Unhooked to Escape to the clear blue yonder —
High up and far-far away

Freed my essence from my breast as
my breast is taken from me
Reduced — no longer there to seduce -
I am less.
Smaller.
Isolated.
Island stated.
Lost and diminished.

Going now — perhaps before Ailsa.
Evaporating
Like a contrail on a high blue cloudless day.

Jackie Swift, Deviot, Austrailia, has published poetry, stories and articles in a range of publications over 20 odd years, plus several unpublished novels. She has won two national writing prizes, one about my experience with breast cancer.

"I am a cancer survivor — breast cancer a few years ago now when, I was 42. The first two poems are based on my own experiences and the third is about a much loved family friend who died suddenly from cancer."

Thom Tammaro
A Dream of My Father

> My young son is still up, reading.
> Suddenly he bursts out laughing,
> And all the sadness of the
> Twilight of my life is gone.
>   Lu Yu, 12th Century

I am walking down Center Avenue
Hat on, looking as I do now.
How little I've changed
Even in my dream.
I am no stranger here,
The son who made you cry.
It is not winter or spring.
It is no season here.
I turn up 12th Street,
Walk until the road ends,
Then stand at the bottom of the hill.
At the top, the pink house you built.
No matter how hard I try, I can't climb
The sixty-seven steps to the top.
You see how I remember small details?
I know you are in the house, dying.
We can't see each other.
You don't know I'm here/there.
My body feels your pain.

Like Lu Yu, I want you
To walk out some night,
See how high the moon is,
Let the damp wind ruffle your coat.
I want you to come back
And hear me laugh.
To make the sadness go away.
Yours. Mine.

Thom Tammaro, Moorhead, MN, teaches at Minnesota State University at Moorhead, where he is Professor of English and teaches in the MFA in Creative Writing program. His poems, essays, reviews and interviews have appeared in numerous anthologies and magazines including *American Poetry Review, The Bloomsbury Review, Chicago Review, The Chronicle of Higher Education, College Composition and Communication, The Emily Dickinson Journal, Great River Review, Midwest Quarterly, North Dakota Quarterly, Quarterly West, South Dakota Review, Spoon River Quarterly, The Sun: A Magazine of Ideas, University of Windsor Review,* and *VIA: Voices in Italian Americana.* He is the author of two full-length collections of poems, *Holding on for Dear Life* and *When the Italians Came to My Home Town,* a finalist for a Minnesota Book Award, and a chapbook, *Minnesota Suite.* He co-edited *To Sing Along the Way: Minnesota Women Poets from Pre-Territorial Days to the Present* (New Rivers Press, 2006); *Visiting Frost: Poems Inspired by the Life and Work of Robert Frost* (2005); *Visiting Walt: Poems Inspired by the Life and Work of Walt Whitman,* a finalist for a Minnesota Book Award (2003); and *Visiting Emily: Poems Inspired by the Life and Work of Emily Dickinson* (2000), winner of a Minnesota Book Award, all published by the University of Iowa Press. He is also the co-editor of *Imagining Home: Writing from the Midwest* and *Inheriting the Land, Contemporary Voices from the Midwest* (University of Minnesota Press), winners of Minnesota Book Awards. He has also edited *Remembering James Wright* by Robert Bly (1991) and *Roving Across Fields: A Conversation with William Stafford and Uncollected Poems 1942-1982* (1983).

"This poem is about a son witnessing his father's death by cancer."

Tammi Truax
Fruit Basket Phobia

When your husband dies young
people bring you fruit,
or have it delivered
by a stranger.

And soon you are left — alone,
with the profoundly painful problem
of still having
a dead husband,

that you have to bury, in the ground,
and little children to care for
who now are crying over something
you can never ever fix,

and a kitchen full
of slowly decomposing fruit
bringing horrifying little fruit flies
into your home, your life.

Silent winged harbingers
of the rotten tomrrows
yet to come.

Tammi Truax, Portsmouth, NH, has published in *The Portsmouth Herald* and *The Poet's Touchstone*.

"I was widowed to cancer at age 38, and also lost my mom and mother-in-law to it within the following 4 years. I have also had several health scares of my own, but so far remain cancer free."

Bill Vernon
Guinea Pig

Stroking Monica's back
the same way you stroked
your cancer-ridden father,

you think, she's not
human, and stop.
Yet moving one floor above it,

you hear the thrashing
in sawdust, the vocalizing too,
not her normal squeak
for water, but grunts of
Ooh! Something's wrong! Help!

So you remember
how a neighbor box-trapped
tomato-eating squirrels
and let a car's exhaust
do the trick.

How hunters snap
the neck of wounded rabbits.
How farmers wring off
the heads of live chickens.
Or use a hatchet.

Bill Vernon, Dayton, OH, a retired college English professor, has four published poetry chapbooks, and individual poetry and fiction in online and hard-copy journals in *Aethlon, Fourth River* and *NEBO*. His novel *OLD TOWN* will be published by *Five Star Mysteries*.

"I was thinking of both of my parents in the cancer-related poems I submitted. My father died of leukemia. My mother had but recovered, miraculously, given a few months only to live by her physician, from lymphoma."

Dorit Weisman
Naomi Paints

Naomi paints my body with a brush
And red strips of light are on the machine, on the ceiling.

Reflections. Inside my body cells are being
Killed. Renewal processes stop.

Radioisotopes are being radiated, attacking.
Your voice, Naomi, is pleasant

I am lying down in a big temple on an elevated bed
A machine sends vibes into my body

Like a boat engine going away
On a river in Turkey

Once the door is closed we are alone in the room, the machine and
me.
The metal giant turns around its axis

First to my right, a steady hum
Then to my left, a jerky hum.

Let me move you,
Don't even think of helping me.

I let you, Naomi, I let you
I am quiet, only those cells I am determined not to

Dorit Weisman, Jerusalem, Israel, won the Prime-Minister Prize for Israeli writers, 2003. She was the winner of the Yehuda-Amichi Prize for Poetry, 2003; Her exhibition of poems written during cancer therapy was titled, *Where Did You Meet Cancer*. Her poetry books include *Where Did you meet the Cancer* (Carmel

Publishing House, 2006); *Dancing Csardas With You — Poems: Parting From Mother* (*Even-Choshen Publishers*, 2005); *What Do the Baobab Trees Stand For? — Poems From the Southern Hemisphere* (*Even-Choshen Publishers*, 2003); and many others. Her work is translated by Rachel Yakobovitz.

"In March 2002, after a routine mammography, I was told by a doctor that I have a malignant tumor in my left breast. I was operated on to remove the tumor; received radiation and took a medicine that had very severe side-effects. I recovered. The cancer was a turning point for me. I changed my life completely. I am retired and I am dedicating my life completely to creativity—writing poems and fiction, translating, painting, playing the piano. My volume of poems about my healing process (*Where Did You Meet the Cancer*) reflects my fight with my cancer, my success, my hope. It reveals great positive powers of life."

Patricia Wellingham-Jones
Don't Turn Away

We've had our drinks, our plural dates,
talked about everybody we ever knew.
Shared many kisses, the last of them
deep, rubbed aching bodies
against each other.
Now you want to undress me.
I don't know if I can bear it.
Sometime back, I told you
about the phony lump in my bra.
But soon, your warm hands will slide
along my ribs, unhook the flesh-colored lace,
gather me in for a long hug. Then,
when you step back and run your eyes
over my one nipple, across the dented
healing slash, up to my face,
will I see on your skin
the ripple of revulsion, a strained smile,
the cooling of heat?
Or will the softness in your eyes
bring tears of thanks to mine
as chest hair tickles scar tissue
and the northern lights flash?

Patricia Wellingham-Jones, Tehama CA, psychology researcher and writer/editor
is a three-time Pushcart Prize nominee. Her published work includes *HazMat
Review*, *Red River Review*, *Rattlesnake Review*, *Phoebe*, *A Room of Her Own*,
Centrifugal Eye, *Ibbetson Street Press* and *Niederngasse*. Chapbooks include *Don't
Turn Away: Poems About Breast Cancer* (PWJ Publishing), *Apple Blossoms at Eye
Level* (Poets Corner Press), *Voices on the Land* (Rattlesnake Press), and *Hormone
Stew* (Snark Publishing). Her collection of caregiver poems, *End-Cycle*, is the
winner of Palabra Productions Chapbook Contest, 2006. She has a 26-article
series called "*Getting Published*" archived on *Long Story Short* www.longstoryshort.
us has a monthly poetry column in *East Valley Times* and has been featured poet

in several journals. Patricia is also publisher of PWJ Publishing and edits and produces books by invitation. Her website is www.wellinghamjones.com.

"I had a mastectomy almost 7 years ago, doing great, thanks. Also spent last year helping our regional cancer center develop a writing program for survivors, patients, family, friends; it's quite successful now and very rewarding."

"I certainly enjoy every day/minute (well, usually) of my life. Cancer is a great wake-up call!"

Patricia Wellingham-Jones
Suppose the Owl Calls My Name

> In Native American lore, the talking bird
> calls the name of the person about to die.

My friend celebrated five years and safety
with a champagne brunch and request:
guests must wear red to give courage,
affirm life. We showed up with flowers
and scarlet, from g-string to tee shirt
to long velvet gown.

Some months later we went into shock
as she lost her second breast.
Raged and wept, built up her spirits
with gifts of red.

Today I lie awake just before dawn,
focus on the owls calling along the creek.
My ears strain to make sense of soft mutters.
On these mornings of dark questions
I rethink my day's clothes, haul out the red socks,
yank myself up.

The owls, incoherent, subside into sleep.

Patricia Wellingham-Jones
Pictures for an Artist

You need to know
what a real mastectomy
looks like so you can draw
that nude I commissioned. So,
after strong English tea
has got us in the mood,
I strip to my skin
on the sun-filled, tree-lined
deck. You snap pictures
of that scar: the dented skin
over ribs, riffled puckers
over sternum, the bluish cast
of flat skin stretching
both sides of the scar.
You click the shutter.
We laugh. I lounge
on a wood bench dotted
with bird droppings.
Drape an antique silk shawl—
soft green with foot-long fringe—
across my jean-clad, naked-
breast body. I don't care
what happens to photos,
drawings, reputation,
if someone calls the cops.
I just sprawl there
in late afternoon warmth,
silk whispering over
my flesh, the one taut
nipple, draw a deep breath,
forget the camera
and smile.

Patricia Wellingham-Jones
Walk of the One-Breasted Women

A strange congregation,
these warrior women
creating our own modern myth.
Feet clunky in Reeboks
we march down Main Street,
less interested in destination
than in being.
Hairless heads helmeted
in turbans, wigs and baseball caps
(full heads of hair
follow rites of passage).
Not all are one-breasted.
Some have no breasts, others
a sad little half, or large pinch
taken out of the fullness.
Each carries a shield,
tiny ribbon loop in pink
pinned on the front of her shirt.
Most have taken poison
to drive out the invader, all
live with the sense of time racing.
On this day we join together,
pool our ages, strength,
our hearts. Watch as people
on the streets join in.
By the end of the walk
we're all laughing with joy,
send a glow of hope heavenward
in a cloud wrapped with pink.

Patricia Wellingham-Jones
The Flow

I sit in my corner window,
watch the neighbor's irrigation
water pour over the dike, spill down the little slope
to flood the land, his and parts of ours.
It washes bugs to the surface where robins
and starlings feast in the sun
then flows, a shimmering sheet,
back to the river, delta, sea.
Mixed and blended, each droplet
merges with the others into something new.
I watch the neighbor's irrigation
and think of my recent diagnosis.
Consider the water's ending, beginning—
the passage of one small drop,
the course of one small life.

Martin Wilitts, Jr.
The Hospital Approaches As a Prescription of Pain

I watch as a sparrow in the field. I watch
the rows of fences marking the miles to the hospital.

She responds: *Please go away.*
She is right. There is nothing
I can do except watch as a field of sparrows.

The miles of loneliness taste like a radish.
If you blank out the pain, whitewash the screams,
it would not make anything better.

It will get better, I promise. She knows a row of lines
when she sees them, even if it darts over fields as a sparrow.

Martin Wilitts, Jr., Norwich, NY. He has produced a fifth chapbook, *Falling In and Out of Love* (Pudding House Publications, 2005), an online chapbook "*Farewell—the journey now begins*" www.languageandculture.net, 2006), and a full-length book of poems with his paper artwork *The Secret Language of the Universe* (March Street Press, 2006). His new chapbook *Lowering Nets of Light* (Pudding House Publications, 2007) which includes his poems about cancer. He is co-editor of www.hotmetalpress.net and the judge of its 2007 poetry chapbook contest. He won the 2007 Chenango County Council of the Arts Individual Artist Grant, which is funding this project.

"This is all because of Francis Willitts."

Martin Willitts, Jr

A Letter from Karen

(for Carolina Sineni)

Dear Mom,

I am at a better place now
where the room does not darken at sundown
where shrimp boats lower nets of light
where the shoals never rise with fists
where the beach is never crowded
as the lighthouse beacon swings over the land
casting light in all directions
where the rocking chair has a cushion
as I knit from endless yellow skeins of yarn
where everything reminds me of postcards
the dirt road ambles by the front picket fence
lined with pansies and yellow irises,
where they still deliver bottles of milk
where no one needs to lock the door
where everyone smiles
carrying buckets of conversation
where no one grows tired of giving greetings
wanting to invite you to visit
tasting homemade cookies still warm
where the hard work never begins or ends

On a clear day, I can see you across the fields
in the kitchen baking pies,
worrying the dough with your fists,
the apples peeled as wet eyes, the apron
smudged with flour, your dress on a line
flapping as it waves hello, your future husband
pruning tomato plants, smelling like mulch.

Your life is a poem needing revision.
You take each word in your life and shake it
as cinnamon. When you do this, I know your pain
as clear as the timer on the oven, or the peels in the basket,
or the sugar on your cheeks, or the warmth of the kitchen
as you bake as if your life depended on it.

Slow down, enjoy that comfort.
I am there with you, reciting the recipe.
I am with you setting the temperature.
When you slice that pie, I will help you with the knife.
When the dishes need cleaning, leave them for me.
Leave them for tomorrow. Go into the living room
and compose reams of language out of his tomatoes.

At night, turn out the light, lie as spoons,
hold him like you held me when I was afraid of the dark,
think about the fact that it is always light here
and there is no more darkness to fear.

Martin Willitts, Jr.
Captive

(Based on a picture and title by Florin Mihai)

A twig of willow deposited in tap water
with its stem a great promoter of healing.

Change is possible from this drink
releasing the hexagon bolt strangling my aorta

allowing freedom from depression
to mention your name

your voice
large as spots on the underside

of the wings
of a Tawny Owl butterfly.

I sip from the water, feeling better,
as if from bluebells.

Christopher Woods
The Calf

Dawn, horizon red in the East,
Clouds created a low ceiling
For the speckled crimson sky.
I walked my retriever
On his constitutional.

Across a neighbor's fence,
I watched the cows,
A procession of sorts,
Coming up from the grove.
One by one they marched.
Coming up the rear was a brown cow,
And, trying to keep pace with her,
A baby calf born in the night.

My wife and I had come to the country
For the weekend, to await pathology results.
She had breast cancer surgery a few days before.
Our lives were in a kind of upheaval,
Not knowing what might happen next.
For the first time, I had thought about fragility
In a new way, how things might end.
I had no idea what the news might be.

Then, seeing this calf, still wet
And struggling on its floundering legs
To keep up with its mother,
I was struck by the cycle of all of us.
For a brief moment, the calf looked at me.
I knew I was the first human
The calf had ever seen.
He studied me for a moment,

Showed a primal kind of recognition,
Then looked away, back to its mother.
And I looked away, into the distance,
Unsure where and how it might be.

Christopher Woods, Houston, Texas, has a prose collection, *Under a Riverbed Sky*.

"My wife, Linda is the cancer victim — breast cancer, specifically. She is currently in chemotherapy."

Anne Harding Woodworth
Old Woman, Pre-op

Before the ride to the hospital
I'll spray "Eternity" behind my ears
that remember kisses on front porches.
I'll wear my silver bangles from those years,
so I can clang like a priest's bells
down the corridor, waking the ICU.

I'll put blue on my eyelids,
purple-brown on my lips,
brush my cheeks pink the way they were
in winter's night-time sledding,
when we screeched throaty noises
into the freezing snow-sky,

while our parents in warm nearby houses
pretended to be compatible after the war,
thought about moving to better neighborhoods,
acquiring Oldsmobile Eighty-Eights,
and how one of these days
they'd teach us to say our prayers.

When the knife cuts into my flesh,
I'll be thinking about a girl, tumor-free.
And no one will say
that I don't smell ravishing enough for a kiss,
that I am not colorful,
that bell-like I don't call out still skyward.

Anne Harding Woodworth, Cedar Mountain, NC. She is the author of
two books of poetry and a chapbook. Her poetry and essays are published or
forthcoming in U.S. and Canadian journals, such as *TriQuarterly*, *Painted Bride
Quarterly*, *Green Mountains Review*, *Antigonish Review*, and *Poet Lore*. She
has have an MFA in poetry from Fairleigh-Dickinson University, is past chair

and current member of the Poetry Board at the Folger Shakespeare Library, Washington, D.C.

"Enclosed here are two poems based on others affected by cancer. The second poem is about one of my closest friends."

Anne Harding Woodworth
Looking for Oncology

[Go to the end of the ramp, through the double door, turn left down
the hall, turn right, second door on left.]

Thanks.
I'm going,
an endoscope,
going down
a throat.
Turn right.
Can smell it,
spongy fungal,
mollusk.
Taste it, too,
bloody, salty,
yeast-like, warm.
Can't find it.
Widen the lens,
It's dark.
I'm panicking,
afraid of foul-mouthing,
of giving up,
inside walls thick with years
of coatings, epithelia.
The f-stop is stuck.
Turn on a light,
turn right.
The door, please,
will somebody
show me
the door.

Alessio Zanelli
Mr. Palmer

Mr. Palmer gathered wood
and resold it just to keep
the pot boiling—sometimes
had the luck to gather
even iron and copper.
When not engaged with the bottle,
he also liked to incise wood.
He carved—at times inlaid—walnut,
briar, oak, mahogany and cherry,
if only someone brought him some.
He skillfully handled
chisels and gouges—
when able to retrieve them.
He used to carve pieces of art
for next to nothing or a cig,
just as an opponent artist's
tools—the smoke and wine indeed
he never ceased to love so much—
inchmeal furrowed his face, stomach
and lungs till demise.
Mr. Palmer ultimately let cancer make
himself his acknowledged masterpiece.

Alessio Zanelli, Cremona, Italy, has long adopted English as his writing language and has published widely in literary magazines around the world including the UK, *Aesthetica*, *Dream Catcher*, *Orbis*, *Other Poetry*, *Poetry Nottingham* and *Pulsar*. He is the author of three collections, most recently *Straight Astray*, and a featured author in the *2006 Poet's Market*.

"The poem is about a real person who lived in my village and died of cancer, and was first published in *Poetry Monthly* (Nottingham, UK). It was also included in my collection *Straight Astray* (Troubador, UK, 2005). Moreover, and curious to say, a picture of the Mr. Palmer (whose real name was Palmiro), which I myself shot in 1989, was used as the cover image of the Winter 2002/2003 issue of *Poetry Review* (London)."

www.ingramcontent.com/pod-product-compliance
Lightning Source LLC
Chambersburg PA
CBHW072135020426
42334CB00018B/1808